Occupational Therapy Assessment Tools: An Annotated Index— Second Edition

Ina Elfant Asher, MS, OTR/L

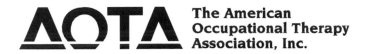

AOTA The American
Occupational Therapy
Association, Inc.

Table of Contents

Parachek Geriatric Rating Scale
Performance Assessment of Self-Care Skills, version 3.1 (PASS)
Scorable Self-Care Evaluation
Structured Observational Test of Function (SOTOF)
        See also: Canadian Occupational Performance Measure (COPM)
                Comprehensive Occupational Therapy Evaluation (COTE)
                Developmental Programming for Infants and Young Children
                Functional Assessment Rating Scale (FAST)Functional Performance
                Record (FPR)
                Occupational Performance History Interview (OPHI)
                Pediatric Evaluation of Disability Inventory (PEDI)
                Routine Task Inventory (RTI-2)
                Scales of Independent Behavior (SIB)
                Vulpe Assessment Battery (VAB-R)

Vocational Assessments

Adult Skills Evaluation Survey for Persons with Mental Retardation (ASES)
APTICOM®*+
Geist Picture Interest Inventory
Jacobs Pre-Vocational Assessment (JPVA)
McCarron-Dial System (MDS)*+ and Perceptual–Motor Assessment for Children (PMAC)*+
Reading-Free Vocational Interest Inventory
Valpar Component Work Sample Series and Dexterity Modules*+
Vocational Interest, Temperament and Aptitude System® (VITAS)
Vocational Adaptation Rating Scales (VARS)
Vocational Interest Inventory–Revised (VII-R)*
Vocational Research Interest Inventory® (VRII)*
Vocational Transit Aptitude Battery®*+
Work Adjustment Inventoroy: Measures of Job-Related Temperament (WAI)
Worker Role Interview (WRI)
        See also: Crawford Small Parts Dexterity Test
                Hand-Tool Dexterity Test
                Jebsen Hand Function Test
                Minnesota Rate of Manipulation Tests (MRMT) and Minnesota Manual
                        Dexterity Test (MMDT)
                Minnesota Spatial Relations Test (MSRT)
                Occupational Role History
                Purdue Pegboard
                Roeder Manipulative Aptitude Test
                Street Survival Skills Test (SSST)

Play Assessments

Children's Playfulness Scale (CPS)
Play History
Play Observation
Preschool Play Scale, Revised
Test of Playfulness (ToP)+

Transdisciplinary Play-Based Assessment (TPBA)

Leisure Assessments

Activity Index: Activity Patterns and Leisure Concepts Among the Elderly (Nystrom) and Occupational Behavior and Life Satisfaction Among Retirees (Gregory)
Interest Checklist
Leisure Activities Blank
Self-Assessment of Leisure Interests
See also: Assessment of Occupational Functioning (AOF)
Canadian Occupational Performance Measure (COPM)
Geist Picture Interest Inventory: Revised
National Institutes of Health Activity Record (ACTRE)
Occupational Case Analysis Interview and Rating Scale (OCAIRS)
Occupational Performance History Interview (OPHI)
Volitional Questionnaire

Performance Components

Sensory Awareness and Sensory Integration Assessments

DeGangi–Berk Test of Sensory Integration
Infant/Toddler Symptom Checklist: A Screening Tool for Parents
McGill Pain Questionnaire (MPQ)
Pain Apperception Test (PAT)
Sensory Integration and Praxis Tests (SIPT)*+
Sensory Integration Inventory–Revised–for Individuals with Developmental Disabilities
Test of Sensory Function in Infants (TSFI)

Perceptual and Visual–Motor Integration Assessments

Behavioural Inattention Test (BIT)
Chessington O.T. Neurological Assessment Battery (COTNAB)
Developmental Test of Visual Motor Integration, 3rd Revision (VMI)
Developmental Test of Visual Perception, 2nd Edition (DTVP-2)*
Hooper Visual Organization Test (VOT)
Jordan Left–Right Reversal Test, Third Revised Edition
Minnesota Spatial Relations Test (MSRT)
Motor-Free Visual Perception Test–Revised (MVPT-R) and Motor-Free Visual Perception Test–Vertical (MVPT-V)
OSOT Perceptual Evaluation, Revised
Rivermead Perceptual Assessment Battery (RPAB)
Test of Visual–Motor Skills (TVMS) and Test of Visual-Motor Skills: Upper Level Adolescents and Adults (TVMS:UL)
Test of Visual–Perceptual Skills (TVPS) and Test of Visual-Perceptual Skills (Non-Motor): Upper Level Adolescents and Adults (TVPS:UL)

Infant and Child Development (Neuromusculoskeletal/Developmental) Assessments

Assessment of Preterm Infants' Behavior (APIB)+
Bayley Infant Neurodevelopmental Screener (BINS)
Bayley Scales of Infant Development, 2nd Edition (BSID-II)
Behavior Rating Instrument for Autistic and Other Atypical Children, 2nd Edition (BRIAAC)+

Callier-Azusa Scale
Clinical Observations of Motor and Postural Skills (COMPS)
Denver II[+]
Developmental Programming for Infants and Young Children
Erhardt Developmental Prehension Assessment (Revised) (EDPA) and Short Screening Form
(EDPA-S)
Erhardt Developmental Vision Assessment (Revised) (EDPA) and Short Screening Form
(EDPA-S)
FirstSTEP Screening Test for Evaluating Preschoolers
Hawaii Early Learning Profile, Revised (HELP®)*
The INFANIB
Milani–Comparetti Motor Development Screening Test, Third Edition Revised
Miller Assessment of Preschoolers
NCAST (Nursing Child Assessment Satellite Training) Feeding and Teaching Scales[+]
Neonatal Behavioral Assessment Scale (2nd Edition) (NBAS)[+]
Neurological Assessment of the Preterm and Full-Term Newborn Infant
Newborn Individualized Developmental Care and Assessment Program (NIDCAP)[+]
Pediatric Evaluation of Disability Inventory (PEDI)*
Quick Neurological Screening Test (QNST)
Vulpe Assessment Battery-Revised (VAB-R)
See also: Developmental Test of Visual Motor Integration (VMI)
Evaluation Tool of Children's Handwriting (ETCH)
Mullen Scales of Early Learning
Peabody Developmental Motor Scales (PDMS)
Sensory Integration Inventory-Revised
Test of Gross Motor Development (TGMD)
T.I.M.E. Toddler and Infant Motor Evaluation

Motor Assessments

Bruininks–Oseretsky Test of Motor Proficiency
Children's Handwriting Evaluation Scale (CHES) and Children's Handwriting Evaluation
Scale for Manuscript Writing (CHES-M)
Crawford Small Parts Dexterity Test
Dueul's Test of Motor Apraxia
Evaluation Tool of Children's Handwriting (ETCH) (Manuscript: ETCH-M and Cursive:
ETCH-C)
Functional Test for the Hemiparetic Upper Extremity
Hand-Tool Dexterity Test
Jebsen Hand Function Test
Minnesota Handwriting Test (MHT)
Minnesota Rate of Manipulation Tests (MRMT) and Minnesota Manual Dexterity Test (MMDT)
Motor Assessment Scale (MAS)
Peabody Developmental Motor Scales (PDMS)
Purdue Pegboard
Roeder Manipulative Aptitude Test
Sensorimotor Performance Analysis (SPA)
Test of Gross Motor Development (TGMD)
T.I.M.E. Toddler and Infant Motor Evaluation

See also: Assessment of Motor and Process Skills (AMPS)
      Behavior Rating Instrument for Autistic and Other Atypical Children (BRIAAC)
      Clinical Observations of Motor and Postural Skills (COMPS)
      Erhardt Developmental Prehension Assessment (EDPA)
      Milani–Comparetti Development Screening Test
      Mullen Scales of Early Learning
      Valpar Dexterity Modules
      Vocational Transit Aptitude Battery
      Vulpe Assessment Battery-Revised (VAB-R)

Cognitive Assessments

Allen Cognitive Level Test (ACL)
Allen Diagnostic Module (ADM)*
The Autobiographical Memory Interview (AMI)
Bay Area Functional Performance Evaluation (BaFPE) (Second Edition)
Blessed Dementia Rating Scale
Clinical Dementia Rating (CDR)
Cognitive Adaptive Skills Evaluation (CASE)
Cognitive Assessment of Minnesota (CAM)
Cognitive Performance Test (CPT)
Contextual Memory Test (CMT)
Doors and People
Global Deterioration Scale (GDS), including Brief Cognitive Rating Scale (BCRS) and Functional Assessment Staging (FAST)
Goodenough–Harris Drawing Test
Leiter International Performance Scale+
Loewenstein Occupational Therapy Cognitive Assessment (LOTCA)
The Middlesex Elderly Assessment of Mental State (MEAMS)
Mini-Mental State (MMS)
Mullen Scales of Early Learning*
Peabody Picture Vocabulary Test–Revised (PPVT)
Prospective Memory Screening (PROMS)
Rivermead Behavioural Memory Test (RBMT)
Routine Task Inventory (RTI-2)
Severe Impairment Battery (SIB)
Short Portable Mental Status Questionnaire (SPMSQ)
Test of Everyday Attention (TEA)
Test of Orientation for Rehabilitation Patients (TORP)
See also: Assessment of Motor and Process Skills (AMPS)
      Functional Behavior Profile (FBP)
      Developmental Programming for Infants and Young Children
      Kitchen Task Assessment (KTA)
      SHORT-CARE

Psychological Assessments

Internal/External Scale
Locus of Control for Children

Personal Value Scales

Philadelphia Geriatric Center Morale Scale

Piers–Harris Children's Self-Concept Scale

Self-Esteem Scale

SHORT-CARE (as derived from CARE, Comprehensive Assessment and Referral Evaluation)[+]

Stanford Preschool Internal–External Scale (SPIES)

Tennessee Self-Concept Scale—Revised (TSCS)*

Volitional Questionnaire (2nd Edition)

> See also: Comprehensive Occupational Therapy Evaluation (COTE)
> Behavior Rating Instrument for Autistic and Other Atypical Children, (BRIAAC)
> Developmental Programming for Infants and Young Children
> Functional Performance Record (FPR)
> Geriatric Rating Scale/Stockton Geriatric Rating Scale
> McGill Pain Questionnaire (MPQ)
> Occupational Questionnaire
> Pediatric Evaluation of Disability Inventory (PEDI)
> Work Adjustment Inventory: Measures of Job-Related Temperament (WAI)
> Worker Role Interview (WRI)

Social Skills and Role Performance Assessments

Adolescent Role Assessment

Assessment of Communication and Interaction Skills (ACIS)

Occupational Role History

Role Checklist

> See also: Occupational Performance Assessments section
> AAMR Adaptive Behavior Scales
> Bay Area Functional Performance Evaluation (BaFPE) (Second Edition)
> Behavior Stream/Specimen Records
> Behavior Rating Instrument for Autistic and Other Atypical Children (BRIAAC)
> Developmental Programming for Infants and Young Children
> Functional Behavior Profile (FBP)
> Katz Adjustment Scale
> National Institutes of Health Activity Record (ACTRE)
> Pediatric Evaluation of Disability Inventory (PEDI)
> Routine Task Inventory (RTI-2)
> Scales of Independent Behavior (SIB)
> SHORT-CARE
> Social Climate Scales
> Vineland Adaptive Behavior Scales, Revised (VABS)
> Work Adjustment Inventory: Measures of Job-Related Temperament (WAI)
> Worker Role Interview (WRI)

Self-Management and Coping Skills Assessments

AAMR Adaptive Behavior Scale—Residential and Community, Second Edition (ABS-RC:2) and AAMR Adaptive Behavior Scale—School, Second Edition (ABS-S:2)

Coping Inventory

Early Coping Inventory

Katz Adjustment Scale
Scales of Independent Behavior (SIB)*
Street Survival Skills Questionnaire (SSSQ)*
Vineland Adaptive Behavior Scales, Revised (VABS)
> See also: Assessment of Motor and Process Skills (AMPS)
> Assessment of Occupational Functioning (AOF)–Second Revision
> Occupational Case Analysis Interview and Rating Scale (OCAIRS)
> Occupational Performance History Interview (OPHI)
> Routine Task Inventory (RTI-2)
> Vocational Adaptation Rating Scales (VARS)
> Vulpe Assessment Battery–Revised (VAB-R)
> Work Adjustment Inventory: Measures of Job-Related Temperament (WAI)

Performance Contexts

Temporal Aspects/Disability Status Assessments

Disability Questionnaire
National Institutes of Health Activity Record (ACTRE)*
Oswestry Low Back Pain Disability Questionnaire
Sickness Impact Profile (SIP)
> See also: Functional Independence Measure (FIM) and Functional Independence Measure for Children (WeeFIM)
> Pediatric Evaluation of Disability Inventory (PEDI)
> SHORT-CARE

Environmental Assessments

Environmental Response Inventory
Home Observation for Measurement of the Environment (HOME)
Social Climate Scale: Ward Atmosphere Scale (WAS) and Community-Oriented Programs Environment Scale (COPES)
> See also: National Institutes of Health Activity Record (ACTRE)
> NCAST (Nursing Child Assessment Satellite Training) Feeding and Teaching Scales
> Newborn Individualized Developmental Care and Assessment Program (NIDCAP)
> Occupational Case Analysis Interview and Rating Scale (OCAIRS)
> Occupational Performance History Interview (OPHI)
> Vulpe Assessment Battery–Revised (VAB-R)
> Worker Role Interview (WRI)

Additional Resources

References

Index of Publishers

Index of Assessment Tool Authors

Index of Assessment Tool Titles

You Can Help

---

*Indicates primary or accessory use of a computer
+Training of examiner is required or recommended

Preface to the Second Edition

The first edition of this reference book, *An Annotated Index of Occupational Therapy Evaluation Tools*, was highly successful, both as a commercial venture and as a professional resource. Therapists around the country have been enthusiastic about its practical use for clinicians, educators, researchers, and students, and have welcomed the plan for an updated version.

Since the first edition was published, a plethora of research has resulted in the development of new instruments designed by and for occupational therapists. As a result, much of the original material became outdated, while new information and assessment tools were being published monthly. The tremendous expansion in this area, as well as the increased emphasis on accountability of services and documentation, necessitated a second edition. Over 100 new assessments are reviewed in this edition, in addition to many revised editions of previous instruments, offering twice the volume of the original text.

The altered title represents a change in the definition of evaluation and assessment. The Commission on Practice has recently clarified OT terminology regarding the difference between the two terms (*OT Week*, July 13, 1995, p. 10). The following definitions were recommended:

- **Evaluation** shall be used to refer to the process of obtaining and interpreting data necessary for intervention. This includes planning for and documenting the evaluation process and results.
- **Assessment** shall be used to refer to specific tools or instruments used during the evaluation process.

The new title of this edition reflects the current terminology and is more consistent with the language used by other health care professionals.

A second major change in the new edition is a result of the publication of the *Uniform Terminology for Occupational Therapy—Third Edition* (*American Journal of Occupational Therapy*, 1994). The organization of the assessments and the section headings reflect the new categories in the Uniform Terminology outline. This is discussed at greater length in the Introduction that follows, where the outline has been reproduced for the reader's benefit.

The instruments profiled in the first edition have been carefully reviewed for this text. Material that was unpublished, out of print, or otherwise unavailable or outdated has been removed. All other original material has been updated by contacting authors and publishers and by reviewing the literature. The remaining profiles reflect these changes. In addition, nearly 100 new instruments have been reviewed, most of which have been developed over the past 5 years. Due to the unending literature on assessment, this collection, like the first, does not attempt to be exhaustive. The selection does not represent an endorsement by the author or by AOTA, but rather reflects the following criteria: availability, utility, a broad sampling of occupational therapy practice, and a state of instrument development in which procedures are standardized and reliability and validity are documented. In addition, most of the material covered has been recently developed or modified to represent current standards.

The Second Edition follows the same format as the First Edition in order to be easily read and used by the reader. The reader is urged to study or review the revised introductory chapter in order to better use and understand the body of assessment profiles that follow.

Acknowledgments

Occupational Therapy Assessment Tools: An Annotated Index—Second Edition is based on a textbook originally prepared for a course in Occupational Therapy Evaluation Tools at Thomas Jefferson University, College of Allied Health Sciences, in Philadelphia. The inspiration and initial concept belonged to Dr. Ruth L. Shem, EdD, OTR/L, FAOTA, who was then professor and chairperson of the department and wished to provide a resource library of assessment instruments for students and clinicians. I am particularly indebted to the many authors, publishers, and distributors of the instruments contained in this book. They encouraged me by their enthusiasm for the project, by their assistance in clarifying the descriptions, and by their generosity in providing me with many test materials for review. I am grateful to Janice Burke, MA, OTR/L, FAOTA, who served as a sounding board for my ideas and questions. It was my privilege to consult with M. Lawrence Furst, PhD, MPH, who advised me on the Introductory chapter and research terminology. Finally, I am thankful for the enthusiastic support of this project by Fran McCarrey, Ethel Anagnoson, and the staff at the American Occupational Therapy Association, who took my 2-year obsession to its happy conclusion.

About the Author

Ina ("Louie") Elfant Asher, MS, OTR/L earned her baccalaureate degree in occupational therapy from Tufts University and her Master of Science degree from Boston University. She is adjunct faculty in the Department of Occupational Therapy, College of Allied Health Sciences, Thomas Jefferson University in Philadelphia. Her extensive experience includes teaching, research, and clinical practice in the treatment of physical disabilities and dysphagia in both hospital and home care settings. Currently, she is directing the establishment of an extensive lending and resource library of assessment tools at Thomas Jefferson University. The library embodies the work in this text by maintaining a collection of instruments as well as an ongoing file of current literature on assessment tools for clinical use, for research, and for continuing education courses. (For more information, see "You Can Help" at the end of this book.)

Ms. Asher has been widely published in occupational therapy journals and books and has conducted several workshops on the treatment of dysphagia. In this, her latest book, Ms. Asher provides a much needed and one-of-a-kind reference guide to assessment tools.

She resides in Merion, Pennsylvania with her husband and four children.

Introduction

In 1984, the Representative Assembly of the American Occupational Therapy Association (AOTA) issued a statement that indicated as a top priority of practice the development of standardized assessments for occupational therapy (OT) and the promotion of their use by therapists. Responding to this need, the AOTA–AOTF Committee on Standardized Assessments/Evaluations published the Hierarchy of Competencies Relating to the Use of Standardized Instruments and Evaluation Techniques by Occupational Therapists (Maurer et al., 1984). According to the basic competencies defined in that paper, the test user:

- . . . recognizes the importance of using standardized, reliable, and valid instruments whenever such are appropriate . . .
- . . . distinguishes the critical differences between standardized and nonstandardized instruments . . .
- . . . recognizes the need to use standardized instruments according to the instructions given in the test administration manual . . .
- . . . recognizes that using standardized instruments in an unstandardized (or adapted) manner may result in an invalid instrument. (p. 804)

This book is the result of a decade of collecting, reviewing, and summarizing standardized and nonstandardized evaluation instruments applicable to occupational therapy. Nearly 200 profiles are contained in the body of the text and reflect the varied areas of OT practice: pediatrics to gerontology, developmental disabilities and sensory integration to physical disabilities and psychiatry. The profiles are of use to the clinician and student who must choose appropriate tools for clinical practice, to the educator who selects assessment procedures for the classroom, and to the researcher who will find instruments that are designed for research purposes or which will benefit from further investigation.

In addition, "Preparing To Test" contains basic information about standardized and nonstandardized tests, their purposes and uses, as well as their advantages and limitations. This first section is intended to address the basic competencies listed above. Before selecting or administering an assessment procedure, the therapist should know what is already available and how to use it properly. **It is hoped that all those who use this book will take the time to study or review the information in this section.**

Occupational Therapy Assessment Tools: An Annotated Index—Second Edition is intended to be a reference book for all occupational therapists. It is hoped that it will provide a service to therapists by aiding in the selection and appraisal of instruments appropriate for use. Finally, may it serve in the crusade for the development and effective use of standardized tests.

Preparing to Test–An Overview of Theory and Terminology

UNIFORM TERMINOLOGY

The third edition of the Uniform Terminology for Occupational Therapy (1994) "is intended to provide a generic outline of the domain of concern of occupational therapy and is designed to create common terminology for the profession..." (p. 1047). This document categorizes and labels the areas of practice for the profession. The authors acknowledge that the categories can be organized in many ways and reiterate that it "is not meant to limit those in the field, formulating theories or frames of reference" or "limit those who would like to conceptualize the profession's domain of concern in a different manner." Rather, it offers an organizing structure for practitioners and a common language for the profession.

For this purpose, *Occupational Therapy Assessment Tools: An Annotated Index—Second Edition* uses the Uniform Terminology as an organizing principle for the text. The contents do not follow a particular frame of reference or theory, although many of the individual assessments are based on identified theories. The goal of this volume is to present a wide range of assessments applicable to all areas of practice and to a broad range of theoretical models. The Uniform Terminology outline is reproduced for the reader's benefit (see Table 1). For further details, the reader is referred to the next section (How To Use This Book).

As noted in the Preface, the definitions of assessment and evaluation have been revised. Assessment now refers to the specific tools or instruments used during the evaluation process. The following is an elaboration of the overall evaluation process as well as its instrumentation.

WHAT IS EVALUATION?

Evaluation "refers to the process of obtaining and interpreting data necessary for treatment" (Maurer, et al., 1984, p. 803). While testing is one form of gathering data, other methods include observation, interview, and review of records. "A test is a systematic procedure for observing a person's behavior and describing it with the aid of a numerical scale or a category-system" (Cronbach, 1970, p. 26). There are many types or forms a test can take: paper-and-pencil tests, oral tests (including interviews), apparatus tests requiring measuring devices, and performance tests requiring the subject to perform a nonverbal task. Although the purpose of evaluation is to obtain objective or factual and verifiable information about the subject, there is a place for clinical judgment by the evaluator or observer. Sound judgment is the analysis and interpretation of information and based on knowledge, experience, and nonverifiable observation. Combined, the objective and subjective sources of information serve to corroborate each other in formulating conclusions.

PURPOSE OF EVALUATION

The primary purpose of evaluation is to obtain accurate information about the subject at a given moment and in a given situation. The results are then applied to practical use: to establish a baseline of performance for later comparison, to measure progress and compare to earlier and/or later measures, to predict future performance in the measured area, to identify or measure specific traits or behaviors, and to identify other traits and behaviors that cause or accompany those measured. Thus,

Table 1

UNIFORM TERMINOLOGY FOR OCCUPATIONAL THERAPY
THIRD EDITION OUTLINE

I. Performance Areas	II. Performance Components	III. Performance Contexts

I. Performance Areas

A. Activities of Daily Living
  1. Grooming
  2. Oral Hygiene
  3. Bathing/Showering
  4. Toilet Hygiene
  5. Personal Device Care
  6. Dressing
  7. Feeding and Eating
  8. Medication Routine
  9. Health Maintenance
  10. Socialization
  11. Functional Communication
  12. Functional Mobility
  13. Community Mobility
  14. Emergency Response
  15. Sexual Expression
B. Work and Productive Activities
  1. Home Management
    a. Clothing Care
    b. Cleaning
    c. Meal Preparation/Cleanup
    d. Shopping
    e. Money Management
    f. Household Maintenance
    g. Safety Procedures
  2. Care of Others
  3. Educational Activities
  4. Vocational Activities
    a. Vocational Exploration
    b. Job Acquisition
    c. Work or Job Performance
    d. Retirement Planning
    e. Volunteer Participation
C. Play or Leisure Activities
  1. Play/Leisure Exploration
  2. Play/Leisure Performance

II. Performance Components

A. Sensorimotor Component
  1. Sensory
    a. Sensory Awareness
    b. Sensory Processing
      (1) Tactile
      (2) Proprioceptive
      (3) Vestibular
      (4) Visual
      (5) Auditory
      (6) Gustatory
      (7) Olfactory
    c. Perceptual Processing
      (1) Stereognosis
      (2) Kinesthesia
      (3) Pain Response
      (4) Body Scheme
      (5) Right-Left Discrimination
      (6) Form Constancy
      (7) Position in Space
      (8) Visual-Closure
      (9) Figure Ground
      (10) Depth Perception
      (11) Spatial Relations
      (12) Topographical Orientation
  2. Neuromusculoskeletal
    a. Reflex
    b. Range of Motion
    c. Muscle Tone
    d. Strength
    e. Endurance
    f. Postural Control
    g. Postural Alignment
    h. Soft Tissue Integrity
  3. Motor
    a. Gross Coordination
    b. Crossing the Midline
    c. Laterality
    d. Bilateral Integration
    e. Motor Control
    f. Praxis
    g. Fine Coordination/Dexterity
    h. Visual-Motor Integration
    i. Oral-Motor Control
B. Cognitive Integration and Cognitive
  Components
  1. Level of Arousal
  2. Orientation
  3. Recognition
  4. Attention Span
  5. Initiation of Activity
  6. Termination of Activity
  7. Memory
  8. Sequencing
  9. Categorization
  10. Concept Formation
  11. Spatial Operations
  12. Problem Solving13. Learning
  14. Generalization
C. Psychosocial Skills and
  Psychological Components
  1. Psychological
    a. Values
    b. Interests
    c. Self-Concept
  2. Social
    a. Role Performance
    b. Social Conduct
    c. Interpersonal Skills
    d. Self-Expression
  3. Self-Management
    a. Coping Skills
    b. Time Management
    c. Self-Control

III. Performance Contexts

A. Temporal Aspects
  1. Chronological
  2. Developmental
  3. Life Cycle
  4. Disability Status
B. Environmental Aspects
  1. Physical
  2. Social
  3. Cultural

evaluation may be diagnostic, may select or classify individuals into categories (e.g., normal or abnormal, independent or dependent), may assist in research (e.g., what is the morale of the geriatric resident in nonprofit vs. for-profit institutions?), and, perhaps most important, may assist in treatment planning and evaluating the effectiveness of treatment. Finally, evaluation may offer the opportunity for establishing a rapport between therapist and client that will be used throughout the treatment process.

THE EVALUATIVE PROCESS

Barbara Hemphill (1982) defines the evaluative process as "using a specific method to measure essential behaviors in a sequential manner" (p. 3). It begins with obtaining a referral and includes data collection in all areas of functioning: psychological, behavioral, learning, and biological. The results are analyzed to identify the client's strengths and abilities, and determine areas of need or deficiency. The conclusions are then applied to make sounder decisions in planning treatment. The process continues until reevaluation is carried out, using the original testing procedures. At this time, treatment is terminated if the client's needs have been met, or new evaluation procedures are used to determine the reason for lack of progress.

METHODS OF DATA COLLECTION

The following are some methods used individually or in combination to gather information (Fox, 1969, Part III).

- *History:* Examine past information to illuminate a question of current interest.
- *Survey:* Using data collection formats, analyze current information to describe,

compare, or evaluate specific phenomena; ranges from mass survey (e.g., demographic studies) to case study (single or multiple individuals).

- *Experimental:* Evaluate a new condition by controlling or manipulating some element(s) of that condition in order to determine a cause–effect relationship.
- *Observation:* Observe natural phenomena or behaviors and draw conclusions to generate hypotheses or predictions about the results of the behavior (e.g., time sampling involves selecting specific time periods to represent the total observation interval).
- *Questionnaire/Interview:* Collect data from the respondent by written or verbal questioning.
- *Measurement:* Collect data for analysis using an appropriate instrument selected or developed for the purpose, such as paper-and-pencil objective tests, performance tests, work samples, projective techniques, inventories, rating scales, mechanical devices, computer programs, and others.

THE STANDARDIZED INSTRUMENT

The standardized instrument is one format used for data collection. This description can be applied to a number of data-collection methods, such as the standardized interview, standardized observation, or standardized test. Cronbach (1970) describes the standardized instrument as one in which the procedure, apparatus, and scoring are fixed so that the same procedures are followed precisely during each administration of the test. The key is uniformity; to ensure this, the instructions to the examiner and examinee must be sufficiently clear, detailed, and complete. The degree of precision varies, of course, and the examiner may discover ambiguities in scoring criteria (e.g., how to determine a rating of 3 versus 4 on a 5-point scale) or instructions (e.g., what to do if the subject does not understand the written instructions).

The primary purpose for standardizing a test is to establish reliability and validity at as high a level as possible. Once test procedures are standardized, the test must be proven *reliable*. That is, if the test is administered repeatedly to the same or comparable subjects, the results should be the same. Obviously, standardized procedures help to ensure the consistency of test administration. A reliable test must also be shown to be *valid*: The test must measure what it is supposed to measure. Now the focus is on what is being measured, no longer on the measurement process itself. (Garfield, in Hemphill, 1982) Both reliability and validity are essential to a sound test. They are determined by several methods that will be described below. The test user must understand these concepts to appropriately use and interpret standardized tests.

Tests with standardized procedures may have *norms* that indicate what scores are usually earned by representative subjects. Collecting normative data involves administering the text to large numbers of subjects to determine what scores should be expected from a normal group. This allows test users to interpret results of a particular test administration by comparing them with the scores achieved by a comparable group of individuals. The process of collecting this information is costly and arduous. Without it, the usefulness of the test may be questioned.

UNDERSTANDING THE STATISTICAL TERMINOLOGY

Test development and standardization involve research using statistical procedures that are not always understood by the user of the test. Although some procedure manuals offer basic information to explain the process, it often requires careful study to understand the data for just one test. To make sense of the information found in the assessment profiles in this book and to offer an elementary lesson in testing, the reader is provided with basic and simplified statistical terminology and general information on test procedures and interpretation. It is hoped that this will not only facilitate the use of these profiles, but will also aid in the reading and critical review of other test manuals as well. In addition, the reader is referred to the reference list at the end of this section. The definitions and explanations that follow were taken primarily from Cronbach (1970), Freeman (1962), Garfield (Hemphill, 1982), and Tarczan (1972).

Before proceeding to the terminology specifically applicable to test standardization, a few generally applicable terms should be understood. **The clinician needs to know enough about research methodology to check the test results knowledgeably and select wisely. The clinician, as the authority on the evaluation results, must understand how test data support the assessment conclusions.** Few clinicians have formal training in methodology, yet this is the basis of a good evaluation. The reliability and validity of the therapist's conclusions are only as good as the reliability and validity of the instrument.

- *Statistics*. The use of mathematics to collect, order, and interpret a set of empirical data in order to describe its characteristics and/or draw inferences from it. Statistical manipulation allows the examiner to determine whether the results are due to the significant effects of experimental variables or to chance factors.

- *Correlation*. The estimated degree of relationship existing between two variables (such as two test scores, two behaviors, or a test score with a predicted behavior). A correlation does *not* imply that one variable causes another, only that they are associated. The relationship between verbal, nonquantitative variables is expressed as an *association*.
- *Correlation coefficient.* This is the numerical index expressing the degree of relationship between two sets of data. The coefficient may range from -1.00 to +1.00. A correlation of ±1.00 means that we can predict perfectly from one test or property to another. In a positive correlation, for example, the individual will score high (or low) on both tests. A negative correlation means that the same individual will score high on one test and low on the other. A zero (0) correlation means that no relationship is evident (i.e., performance cannot be predicted from the test score). Fox (1969) describes correlations that are from 0 to ±.50 as low , ±.50 to ±.70 as moderate, ±.70 to ±.86 as high, and more than ±.86 as very high. Of course, these values must be evaluated in the context of the variables being correlated. There are several statistical procedures that are used to express correlation; they are *not* numerically identical. The more advanced reader will want to distinguish among these procedures, which are beyond the scope of this text.
- *Level of significance*. This statistical procedure identifies the amount of objectivity of data by determining the probability that chance influences the results. The lower the level, the greater the confidence in the data. In the social sciences, .05 (5%) and .01 (1%) level of significance are commonly used, the latter having the lower risk of error. In other words, the probability of a given result occurring by chance is less than 5 (or 1) out of 100.

Reliability

Any measuring instrument yields a certain degree of imprecision. A test's *reliability* is the degree of accuracy and stability of the test, as determined by repeated administrations of the instrument that consistently yield the same results. In addition to describing how dependable the test is in giving stable results, reliability also describes how free the test is from internal defects that will produce errors in measurement (*internal consistency*). Reliability is increased by well-written procedures and a sufficiently large number of items on which to base the score.

To provide estimates of the precision or consistency of a test, reliability coefficients and standard error of measurement are used:

- *Error of measurement.* This is the difference between the subject's universe score (i.e., the score that perfectly represents all observations of the property being examined for that individual) and the score on one observation. Since no single observation represents the entire person, and test scores vary from one measurement to the next, one must generalize from the single observation. The error of measurement is determined by checking the agreement between subsequent scores.
- *Standard error of measurement (SEM).* This is the statistical estimation of how large the error might be in a single observation or score. The SEM is the element of chance in test scores. It is an important calculation because inconsistencies in testing sessions may otherwise obscure the subject's actual

abilities. The smaller the standard error, the greater the confidence that the sample accurately represents the population. The SEM is favorably influenced by greater reliability of test scores and an optimal test environment.

- *Reliability coefficient.* This is the statistic used to describe the relationship between the subject's scores on subsequent observations or testings. The coefficient tells what percentage of the score variance is not error. The more observations that are made, the more the results agree with the universe score. Perfect agreement = 1.00; thus the closer the coefficient is to 1.00, the more reliable the test.

Methods of determining reliability are described as follows.

- *Test–retest* method assesses the stability by administering the same test a second time to the same subject under the same circumstances. The subject should score the same on the retest. A time interval is necessary between the two testings so the subject will not remember the first answers and reproduce them. Because of the time lapse, factors such as maturation, environment, practice, or health changes may influence the retest. The degree to which the test and retest scores correlate indicates reliability. Freeman (1962) reports on test–retest studies in which the correlation on immediate retesting is .90–.95, with 1-year interval is .85, with a 2-year interval is .80,, and over a 5-year interval is .75–.80. The expected reliability also depends on the nature of the information sought. Fox (1969) suggests that high reliability (above .90) should be expected from fixed data (e.g., job history), above .80–.85 for relatively fixed characteristics (e.g., knowledge), and acceptable levels above .70

for more flexible attitudes and interests. Depending on the statistical methodology used, however, a more rigorous examination of the data may claim higher reliability in spite of a lower numerical coefficient.

- *Interrater reliability* means the test is given to one subject but scored by two or more raters. In this case, reliability is improved by training the raters and by clarifying instructions and scoring criteria. Freeman reports that correlations of .85 to .90 are expected from competent examiners. The more subjectivity (that is, the more personal judgment is required) in the scoring, the lower the reliability is apt to be. *Intrarater reliability*, on the other hand, measures the consistency of judgments made by the same rater over a brief interval. Unlike test–retest reliability, which compares scores over time, intrarater reliability compares rater's judgments or observations (Ottenbacher & Tomchek, 1993).

- *Alternate, or parallel, forms* method uses two equivalent forms of one test administered to one subject on the same occasion with a rest in-between, or with a time interval in between (*delayed alternate forms*). The consistency of the two results are then compared. When the time interval is eliminated, this method has the advantage of avoiding the changing influences at different testings. Developing an equivalent version of the test, however, may require considerable research.

- *Internal consistency* reflects the homogeneity among items within a test (see definition of reliability). Consistency within the total or composite score is determined by dividing the single test into equal halves and comparing the score of one half with the score of the other. The correlation coefficient indicates the strength of association among items, demonstrating that they measure a similar quality. There are several systems for dividing the tests, the most common of which are the *split-half* system, in which the first half of the test is compared to the equivalent second half, and the *even–odd* system, in which the even–numbered items are compared to the odd-numbered items.

The statistical means of determining reliability are not described in this text. In the past several years, more has been written in OT literature about statistical analysis, specifically critiquing the various methodologies employed (refer to Ottenbacher & Tomchek, 1993). There may be confusion and disagreement about terminology, inappropriate methods of data analysis, or weak statistical analysis used. (For example, more stringent statistical methods may yield lower reliability coefficients, which may seem weak but actually indicate stronger reliability.) Specific statistical procedures have not been described in this text, nor have they been differentiated in the brief assessment summaries provided. The advanced reader should refer to the original sources for more thorough investigation.

Validity

A test has validity if it has been shown to actually measure what it purports to measure. Obviously, this is of critical importance in testing. An invalid test may be worthless or misleading. A test is designed for a specific use. Clearly, a valid test that is used in a way it was not intended (e.g., a test for children used with adults, or standardized instructions altered) is no longer valid, and results must be interpreted with caution. Also, a test should be validated for every recommended use. One should not ask whether test X is a valid test, but rather, if test X has been determined valid for the decision that has to be made. If a test is being applied in a new way (e.g., a test for sighted adults being used for the blind), it should be validated for that use. An example of revalidation of a test is the Motor-Free Visual Perception Test, designed for children and currently being restandardized for adults. Finally, a test must be reliable to be valid. A test that is unstable cannot be depended upon for making accurate predictions or decisions.

Terminology related to validity follows.

- *Validity coefficient.* This number, which theoretically may range from 0 to 1.00, is the correlation between the test and the criterion. Calculating validity is frequently a simple correlation between test score and each criterion. "A coefficient of a particular size cannot be specified as signifying or not signifying a satisfactory degree of validity" (Freeman, 1962, p. 100). Any positive coefficient in which there is a small measurement of error has value. Of course, the higher the coefficient, the better, but rarely will it exceed .60 (Cronbach). The particular use of a test will help determine a minimum acceptable value.

There are several types of validity. Most instruments employ more than one type, and the different types may overlap. These are described below.

- *Face validity.* The test *seems* to measure what the author intended it to measure. The test items appear to be related to the variables being tested and relevant to the stated purpose. There is no statistical measurement of face validity, but rather it relies on logic and subjective judgment. (Although the validity of the instrument may seem obvious, it may not be so. As an example, grooming, dressing, and bathing items are clearly relevant to activities of daily living [ADL], but are those categories indicative of all ADL? And is a checklist, via oral interview, a valid means of measuring performance?) This is the weakest type of validity.

- *Content validity*. The items contained in the test, individually and as a whole, represent and adequately sample the domain being examined. Content validity is descriptive rather than statistically determined. It reflects a thorough search of the literature and the opinions of experts in the field. (For example, the ADL checklist described above would be expanded to include sample behaviors from 14 areas after consulting textbooks, other ADL tests, and specialists in the field.)

- *Criterion-related validity*. The test results are compared with outside criteria to determine the degree of agreement between the score and the criterion. The criterion is believed to reflect the same or related concepts. There are two types of criterion-related validity, concurrent and predictive:

  - *Concurrent, or congruent, validity* refers to the extent to which the test results agree with other measures of the same or similar traits and behaviors. For example, test scores are compared to scores on existing valid tests administered at the same time. The criterion may be in the same family, or *congruent* (e.g., ADL checklist scores are compared to two other ADL evaluations known to be valid) or in a different category, or *concurrent* (e.g., correlation of perceptual–motor skills with dressing ability).

  - *Predictive validity* refers to the extent to which test results agree with a future outcome or criterion. A follow-up study of the subject's later performance is required to determine if the original scores predicted later performance. This is the strongest type of validity and is used to make predictions about individuals and their future behavior. (Continuing the example of the ADL checklist, subjects who scored highest in independent performance maintained a more active life style 5 years later than did the low scorers.) This type of validity is especially valuable to clinicians who follow up on treatment effectiveness. *Discriminant analysis* can be used to predict into which of two groups a subject is likely to fall (e.g., neonatal test results may predict which children will be normal versus developmentally delayed at 5 years of age).

- *Construct validity* is based on the theoretical framework of the evaluation, that is, how well the data generated by the test fit with theory or concepts. It gauges the ability of the instrument to measure an underlying trait or hypothesis that is not otherwise directly observable. It is used to validate the theory behind the instrument (ADL checklist may confirm a hypothesis that those who remain independent in self-care activities have a more active social life). It may also distinguish between groups known to behave differently on a given variable. In order to demonstrate construct validity, the test should correlate highly with a similar variable (*convergent validity*) and should not correlate with dissimilar variables (*discriminant validity*) (Anastasi, 1968). There are three parts to construct validity, as described by Garfield (Hemphill 1982): (1) describe the concepts (i.e., constructs) that account for test performance; (2) compose hypotheses that explain the relationships of the concepts; and (3) test the hypotheses. Thus, theories are developed by proposing the hypothesis, testing to verify, and revising based on the new data.

- *Factorial validity* may be considered with construct validity because it can identify the underlying structure of the theoretical construct. Factor analysis isolates elements, or factors, that are believed to constitute a collective ability or function. Thus, traits are isolated and categorized in an attempt to organize empirical data. (The Interest Checklist, for example, uses factor analysis to identify discrete, non–overlapping interests and categorize them.) High factorial validity indicates that the test measures one functional unit to the exclusion of others, as far as possible. This is done by measuring intercorrelations among separate, restricted measures.

THE USE OF TESTS

Test Selection

Choice of an evaluation tool may be based on many factors. Some institutions rigidly define what procedures are to be used, and the same regimen is carried out for every client. Other facilities rely on a set of homegrown and informal forms to be used at the therapist's discretion. Still others rely solely on observation and interview and may even disdain the use of standardized instruments.

In a survey Barbara Hemphill (1982) carried out among occupational therapists working in psychiatry, few clinicians were even familiar with the more than 45 testing procedures published in the *American Journal of Occupational Therapy* at that time. She cautioned that therapists should be able to determine which tools will best evaluate which clients. It would be just as foolish to use all test procedures on every client as it would be to evaluate only one area of behavior.

Any therapist learns that the selection of appropriate evaluation tools depends on a careful consideration of the facts known about the client. Usually, this is based upon personal background, medical history, diagnosis, problems presented, and abilities—as gleaned from records, other professional and family reports, interview, observation, and prescription. Testing is an integral part of data collection, although test results are only one of many sources of information.

Although there may be many good tests for a specific function, the therapist must select the test that best fits the decision to be made. It must suit the examiner's purpose, situation, and restrictions (e.g., time, space, population). Directions should be clear, even when non-standardized tests are chosen.

It bears repeating that **a test must be valid for the situation at hand**. As Cronbach points out, the fundamental basis for choosing a test is validity: whether it can be interpreted soundly and the information gained serves the purpose.

Moreover, if the test seems interesting and sensible, it will be a pleasant experience, increasing the cooperation of the subject and resulting in more valid scores.

The test manual is the best source of information on the test. It gives the test directions, scoring procedures and research findings (though some may gloss over unfavorable evidence). **Some tests require training to**

administer; usually, the publisher will restrict access to these tests to qualified individuals.

Finally, therapists who are otherwise resourceful and adaptive may not take liberties with standardized procedures without invalidating test results. Therefore, test selection should consider the special characteristics of the subject. If a test to identify learning disabilities is not meant for severely handicapped children, another test should be used. Group testing should only be done with tests designed for such use. Otherwise, the examiner is encouraged to conduct a simple follow-up study that would establish validity for this new purpose or, when nonstandardized tests do not clearly delineate the limitations of use, improve the test by standardizing the procedures. (Here is the opportunity this author takes to act as crusader for better standardization of tests!)

Test Administration

Test administration ranges from the simple to the complex and subtle, and the examiner must be properly prepared regardless. Differing levels of preparation are required, from reading the instructions or manual in advance and practicing, to formal training in order to obtain certification or advanced degree. Some test materials are released only to trained and qualified personnel. The untrained user may administer a test incorrectly, misunderstand what the test measures, and reach unsound conclusions (Cronbach), as well as spoil the test for future use with that subject.

It is the examiner's responsibility to elicit the subject's best efforts. Cronbach makes the following recommendations to help the examiner achieve this:

- The examiner must become familiar with the test procedures *in advance*.
- During testing, the examiner must maintain an impartial and scientific attitude to ensure fair testing. No coaxing or hints, whether direct ("that's right—good!") or subtle (frowning at an error) are permitted, but rather, the examiner should show an *interest* (silently) in the subject's progress.
- A positive rapport and general encouragement (as permitted) are used to elicit the subject's best cooperation.

Test conditions may be defined precisely in the test manual. In any testing situation, however, the space provided must have adequate ventilation and lighting, as well as a convenient place to write, if necessary. The subject should be well positioned to see any demonstrations and hear directions clearly. The timing of the evaluation should be favorable, that is, when the subject is alert and attentive. Several consecutive tests should be spaced over time. If this is impossible, a critical attitude should be taken toward the results.

Group testing can be done with subjects who are expected to be able to cooperate with the examiner and the test requirements. In group testing situations, the examiner must proceed promptly and efficiently, while allowing for individual questions. Full attention from the group is necessary before beginning. Directions must always be clear, delivered at an appropriate pace in an audible but polite tone of voice.

Giving directions to the subject is the single most important responsibility of the examiner. In a standardized test, the directions must be exactly as they are provided in the manual— word-for-word, no additions, no changes. When the subject asks a question, it must be answered according to the manual's provisions for explanations. For example, if the instructions provided are inadequate, and the norms are based on the use of those instructions, any other supplementation by the examiner will influence the scores and invalidate the comparison to the original norms.

If the subject does not care about the test results, his or her effort is not adequately measured. The subject must feel encouraged and confident, never shown dissatisfaction by the examiner. There are numerous motivations for taking a test: concern for the score, interest in the task, friendliness of the examiner, obedience to authority, praise, and understanding the purpose and benefit of the test. The examiner should consider these in maximizing the subject's cooperation.

Standards of testing have long been the domain of the American Psychological Association (APA). The APA, with the American Educational Research Association and the National Council on Measurement in Education, has published a small volume describing technical standards for test construction and evaluation, and professional standards for test use (1985). In addition, a chapter is devoted to particular applications, including "for people who have handicapping conditions" (p. 77). It is reiterated here that test claims cannot be generalized to modified circumstances unless the claims are reinvestigated.

Scoring and Interpretation

Early in the chapter, a test was defined as "a systematic procedure for observing a person's behavior and describing it with the aid of a numerical scale or a category system." So far, the systematic procedure has been discussed. Now we come to the means of describing the behavior, or the results of the test. While the examiner may gain a good deal of information about the subject merely by observing his or her efforts and reactions to testing, the results or scores are of primary importance.

Since scoring a test can vary greatly among different scorers, objective methods, such as multiple-choice questions, are used to improve uniformity. Tests requiring judgment in scoring may increase objectivity by providing criteria (e.g., definitions of ratings, sample specimens) to compare with the subject's responses. Sometimes the scoring or interpretation of the scores is highly complex and requires advanced training or use of centralized computer services. Even when the score is a simple sum of correct answers, interpretation should be done carefully. Clinicians may depart from the expected interpretation due to mitigating information about the subject (e.g., left visual neglect influenced performance). For this and similar reasons, test results are not considered in isolation, but rather, are confirmed by other sources of information to form a total picture of the subject.

There are many types of scoring systems (e.g., sum totals, ratings), and a variety of ways to express the scores (e.g., raw scores, profiles, age equivalents). It is necessary to review some basic terminology and statistics involved in scoring. The definitions shown in Table 2 should aid the reader in better understanding the basis for scores and interpretations; they are based on Cronbach, Tarczan, and Fox.

Table 2. Scoring and Statistical Terminology

Presentation of scores

- *Score:* actual numerical results obtained from a group of subjects.
- *Raw Score:* direct numerical report of an individual's test performance. The raw score by itself has little significance until an interpretation is offered (e.g., what does a score of 9 mean?) or unless the test content is exhibited (e.g., stereognosis: (+)coin, (+)key, (-) paper clip.
- *Percentile score:* percent of scores falling below the subject's score.
- *Percentile rank:* percent of group falling below the subject's score (e.g., 65th percentile means 65% of the group is below the subject's raw score of 53). The middle scorer thus becomes 50%, or median, or *typical* performance. The advantage of this method is that it is easy to use and understand, and the subject's performance can be compared to other subjects. The disadvantage is that it does not indicate the distance between scores, but has the effect of equalizing the distances (e.g., there is no way to tell whether the high scorer is 1 point or 20 points above the next score).
- *Profile:* graph showing the subject's performance on a variety of tasks. Different test scores can be presented simultaneously and compared, as can subtest scores of one test to compare component or related traits.

Measures of central tendency

- *Mode:* most frequently appearing score. (It gives no information about the range of scores in the group.)
- *Median:* middle score, 50%, or the number that divides the scores into two equal parts. (It is useful in a small sample because it is not influenced by extreme cases or scores.)
- *Mean:* arithmetic average obtained by adding all scores together and dividing the total by the number of scores. This is the most common measure of central tendency. (It is susceptible to distortion by one or two extreme scores.)

Measures of dispersion

- *Range:* a measure of variability obtained by subtracting the lowest from the highest score. The range includes the lowest and highest scores. It reflects the variability of scores within the sample as well as how far the scores vary from the mean.
- *Standard deviation, or SD:* a numerical index that indicates the degree of dispersion of data, or the spread of the scores. It reflects the variability of scores within the sample as well as how far the scores vary from the mean. It is obtained by averaging the departure of the subject's scores from the group mean. (Square each deviation and average the squares to

continues

Table 2, continued

arrive at the variance of the distribution; standard deviation is the square root of the variance). The smaller the *SD*, the closer the scores cluster to the mean, and subjects do not vary widely in performance. Conversely, the larger the *SD*, the farther the distribution of scores from the mean.

Norms and distributions

For test scores:

• *Frequency distribution:* a manner of treating data in which scores are tallied and arranged graphically in the order of magnitude from the lowest to the highest scores. In this way, the mode, median, and mean can be determined. The frequency distribution is used to condense raw data for case of presentation and understanding.

Example:	**Range of Scores**	**Frequency of Occurrence**
	1	2
	2	4
	3	7
	4 (mode)	12
	5 (median)	11
	6 (mcan)	10
	7	9
	8	8
	9	8
	10	7

• *Normal distribution:* arrangement of scores along a bell-shaped curve characterized by a concentration of scores near the average (or peak of the bell) and symmetrical tapering toward each extreme. This is a frequency distribution in which the mean is center peak and *SD* is the distance from the peak to the beginning of the taper on each side. Thus, 68.3% of the scores will fall within one standard deviation of the mean on either side, 95.4% within two standard deviations, 99.7% within three standard deviations. Scores

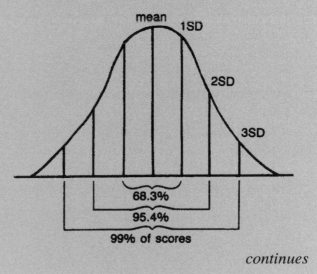

continues

Table 2, continued

are converted to normal distribution for purposes of comparison.

- *Deviation score:* score obtained by subtracting the mean raw score from each raw score. This indicates how far any individual score varies from the mean.
- *Standard score (z-score):* is a method for converting raw scores into a common scale. A standard score scale is based on the mean and *SD* and is calculated by dividing the deviation score by the standard deviation. The z-score can express any raw score as so many standard deviations above or below the mean. If it is known how many standard deviations from the mean a score is, the subject's position vis-a-vis the group can be determined. This is widely used in commercial tests as it is precise and based on very large samples. **Standard scores can be compared because they are based on a common scale**, whereas raw scores are not. Once scores are converted to normal distribution, standard scores can be converted to percentage scores, and vice versa.
- *t-score:* type of standard score adjusted to have a mean of 50 and *SD* of 10. Thus, a score of 70 is two standard deviations above the mean.
- *Stanine scale:* single-digit system in which scores are converted to a scale of 1 to 9, with a mean of 5 and *SD* of approximately 2. This is utilized for its practicality and simplicity.

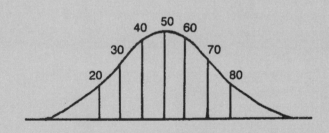

For subjects:

- *Population:* total group of individuals to which the test applies (e.g., congenitally blind adults over age 18).
- *Sample:* group of subjects selected to represent the population in a trial testing. The larger the sample, the better it represents the total population.
- *Random sample:* type of sample in which each individual in the population has the same chance of being selected for the sample as any other.
- *Norms:* test scores of a specified group to which the individual subject's score can be compared. Normal performance is presented on tables that contain percentage scores of the sample. The sample must be defined in order to know if it is representative of the subject. A large size sample is important to adequately represent the range of the population, though size alone does not ensure a satisfactory sample. In some tests, local norms are most useful. Other tests have many norms: different tables for different age ranges, or manual dexterity norms for clerical versus assembly-line workers. It is important to match the subject to the correct norms for the comparison to be valid. (*Note:* norms are not standards; the standard

continues

Table 2, continued

may be that all 8-year-olds read at a third grade level in the U.S., while the norm may be that most 8-year-olds really read at a second grade level. Norms are average or typical scores by testing; standards are goals or objectives that may be above the norm and achieved through further development or improvement [Freeman, 1962].)

Interpretation of scores

- *Norm-referenced test* compares the subject to the population, using the normative tables described above. Thus, scores determine status by comparing the subject's performance to the performance of others (e.g., a disabled worker may compare poorly to norms on a manual dexterity task). Normative data quantify test results and are weighted toward the mean or average of the normative group.
- *Criterion-referenced test* compares the subject's performance to a standard of performance or mastery, rather than to other groups of individuals. Performance criteria use observable behaviors to represent optimal performance (e.g., can the disabled worker dress, eat breakfast, and drive to work in 90 minutes). It is most sensitive to individual gains as the subject is measured against himself or herself. It is also useful in areas such as psychosocial components, such as self-confidence, for which norms are sometimes irrelevant. (Bonder, 1993)

Rasch analysis

The Rasch model (Bruininks et al., 1985; Snyder & Sheehan, 1992) is the basis for rigorous mathematical analysis of item response data used during test development. With Rasch analysis, the measurement properties of a test can be determined. Rasch analysis is used with test items that are unidimensional (measure the same underlying traits), to ensure that items are independent of each other (performance on one item is not influenced by performance on another), and that all items equally discriminate across the range of abilities. Thus, items are analyzed to determine whether they meet these criteria; those that do not are deleted from the test. Resulting test items form an item pool or bank that can easily be converted to parallel forms, or selected to tailor a test to an individual subject.

A significant benefit of Rasch analysis is that person ability and item ability may be represented on a common equal-interval scale. In other words, abilities that would not otherwise be comparable can be plotted on the same scale for scoring. (For example, a preschooler's toileting ability and an adult's time and punctuality habits can both be graded on the Scales of Independent Behavior, and progress in both can be accurately represented by the same scoring system.) Many tests do not have this characteristic, yet treat the score differences as if they were equal interval scales and could be compared. Items are calibrated independently of the subject and can be applied to any individual, eliminating the need for massive normative samples.

Limitations of Testing

Although the use of tests provides a systematic method for obtaining objective and measurable information in an evaluation, test results cannot be the only basis for making decisions about the subject. It bears repeating that test results should be corroborated by other information and observations about the subject. Often mitigating factors must be taken into account when interpreting the results. Each piece of information is confirmed or refuted by other data gathered at the same time; even crude instruments may provide clues for further exploration (Anastasi, "Mental Measurement: Trends," in Mitchell, 1985).

Standardized tests do not allow individualization of procedures beyond the uniform methodology provided. There may not be tests available to accommodate some special needs. In this case, a test may be revalidated for the special purpose or the results treated tentatively enough to allow for the possibility of an invalid test.

Ethical issues must be considered as tests are liable to be abused and misused. Although personality tests are sometimes regarded as an invasion of privacy, *any* interview format may allow the examiner to probe into areas that are not relevant to the trait being measured. Test results may be overgeneralized, and claims may be made that go beyond demonstrated validity (Cronbach, 1970). It is the responsibility of the test developer to avoid cultural bias in the test. Bette Bonder (1985) recommends adopting some of the Ethical Principles for Psychologists. These principles acknowledge the right of clients to know the results of assessments made, the interpretations, and the basis for their conclusions and recommendations.

Furthermore, the American Psychological Association takes responsibility for the security of tests, as well as the individual's rights. Test items that are reproduced and used out of context may destroy the value of the instrument. In addition, psychologists take responsibility for the behavior of others by discouraging use of tests by unqualified personnel. Bonder suggests that occupational therapists protect the instruments, their clients, and themselves by adhering to these ethical principles.

HOW TO USE THIS BOOK

How to Use This Book

This volume contains profiles of instruments that evaluate *performance areas*, *performance components*, and *performance contexts*. The reader is referred to the *Uniform Terminology for Occupational Therapy—Third Edition* outline (see Table 2) for the organizing structure of the chapters. There are occasional departures from the outline for practical purposes. Most notably, infant and child development assessments are collected into a separate chapter, due to the prominence of a pediatric specialty in OT.

The assessments selected for this book were required to demonstrate standardized procedures, evidence of reliability and validity, and results that offered functional interpretation. For example, measuring devices that yield only raw data (e.g., dynamometer) were eliminated. Assessment formats range from interviews to paper-and-pencil tests, checklists to complex performance tasks. Assessments of foundation components, such as range of motion, muscle strength, and sensation are not included. Rather, consistent with the goal of evaluating occupational function, emphasis on such components is placed within a functional context and includes simple skills (e.g., manual dexterity tasks), complex, integrated skills (e.g., household chores), behaviors (e.g., accepts responsibility), and traits (e.g., morale).

The number of evaluations profiled is arbitrary. The list could go on and on. One need only to consult *Tests in Print IV* (Murphy, 1994) to appreciate the vast numbers of published tests available. The selections contained here represent a cross section of occupational therapy practice. Judgments are not made on the quality of the evaluations, and the inclusion or exclusion of instruments does not constitute endorsement of any kind. It is hoped that the descriptive information will provide a sufficient basis for the reader to make selections. Some prominent tests (e.g., of language, intelligence) are not included if it was determined that they are outside the domain of occupational therapy.

The organization of the book is according to topic, so that similar areas of assessment (e.g., vocational, play, and leisure skills) are grouped in proximity. This is designed to facilitate comparisons for the purpose of choosing the best instrument for a particular purpose. Needless to say, there is a great deal of overlap, and some tests measure several areas. Thus, some instruments will be listed in parentheses under additional topics in the Table of Contents. For this reason, there are two indexes for reference: one index of tests listed alphabetically and one index of authors listed alphabetically.

EVALUATION PROFILES

Each of the entries in this book is a summary profile of an instrument. In a few cases, a single profile covers two versions of one instrument or two closely related instruments that are considered together. Each profile describes the instrument under 14 headings. Each of these headings is explained as follows:

- TITLE: The full title of the instrument, as published or as referred to in the source(s) cited, including abbreviations or initials, if applicable.
- AUTHOR(S): Author(s) of the instrument or of the article in which the instrument was first conceived and described.
- FORMAT: indicates form of test, such as observation, rating scale, checklist, etc.
- PURPOSE: what the instrument is intended to measure, as stated by the author, including whether it is designed for clinical and/or

research purposes.

- POPULATION: The group(s) for whom the instrument is intended, including ages, disability, and any limitations or restrictions of use. (A description of the population sample is included when possible.)
- SETTING OR POSITION: Any specifications found in the manual or instructions regarding the test area or the subject.
- MATERIALS OR TOOLS: A summary of items necessary for testing, including or in addition to the test materials or test kit purchased from the publisher.
- METHOD: Test procedures are described in briefest form, sufficient only to give the reader an idea of the process involved; includes, when possible, the number of test items, length of time required, and the scoring method.
- INTERPRETATION: Test yield is described, including the scoring system and meaning of the results (e.g., identifying abilities or impairments for treatment planning).
- RELIABILITY: A summary statement of the reliability data, including type of reliability and the reliability coefficient, if possible, as reported by the test author or manual.
- VALIDITY: A summary statement of the validity research, including type of validity and the validity coefficients, if possible, as reported by the test author or manual.
- SOURCE: How to obtain the test, usually a publisher's address, the reference for the article or book that contains the printed test, or the personal address of the author or sponsoring agency. When available, a date of publication is provided. (Many published tests are available from multiple vendors and distributors, and the reader may check catalogs for the best price.)

- COST: due to constantly changing prices, a cost code is offered instead of a price. Each symbol represents a price range. The lowest price category includes instruments that are printed in published materials available in libraries or universities, or which can be obtained for the cost of postage or reproduction. The code is as follows:

  ¢ = $ 0 to $10
  $ = $11 to $50
  $$ = $51 to $150
  $$$ = $151 to $500
  $$$$ = $501 to $2,000
  $$$$+ = over $2,000

- SAMPLE: When appropriate, a representative item, rating system, or instruction is quoted as an illustration of the test; occasionally, there is no sample given when the test is an unstructured interview or does not use language during test administration.

PERFORMANCE AREAS

Occupational Performance

Assessments

❏ Assessment of Occupational Functioning (AOF)—Second Revision

AUTHORS: Janet Hawkins Watts, MS, OTR, Chestina Brollier, PhD, OTR, FAOTA, David F. Bauer, PhD, and William Schmidt, MS, OTR

FORMAT: Screening tool using semi-structured interview-based rating scale.

PURPOSE: This tool is designed to screen overall occupational function in residents of long-term-care settings. It is based on the model of human occupation and can aid in identifying areas for further assessment and treatment and for discharge planning.

POPULATION: Physically disabled and/or psychiatric patients or residents in long-term-care settings. The authors suggest AOF need not be limited to this setting. (Sample consisted of 83 subjects, ages 60 or older, from a psychiatric hospital, a long-term-care facility for the physically disabled, and a group of people living independently in the community.)

SETTING OR POSITION: Not prescribed.

MATERIALS OR TOOLS: Interview schedule and rating scale; pencil.

METHOD: The AOF consists of two parts. The first, a semi-structured interview schedule, addresses each component of the three subsystems of human function (according to the model of human occupation): volition, habituation, and performance. The second part provides a 5-point scale to rate each of the six model components (values, personal causation, interests, roles, habits, and skills) based on the interview data. The subject completes an additional page with a brief questionnaire on school and job history. A total score ranging from 6 to 30 is obtained by adding component scores. The administration takes fewer than 30–40 minutes.

INTERPRETATION: The test yields a summary profile of occupational function. Items rated with 1–3 may suggest the need for further in-depth evaluation of that area. Interpretation of the total score is not offered, except for use in concurrent validity studies.

RELIABILITY: Interrater reliability of total scores was .78. Test–retest reliability of total scores (14- to 21-day interval) ranged from .70–.90. Item correlations with total score were good (between .70 and .94). Interviewers must be experienced and familiar with the theoretical model to use the AOF and derive meaning from it.

VALIDITY: Content validation based on consultation with experts and adherence to the model yielded the revised version. Concurrent validity is based on expected negative correlations with Life Satisfaction Index-z, with mixed results in correlations with Geriatric Rating Scale. Finally, AOF scores distinguished between the healthy (community) and institutionalized groups.

SOURCES: Watts, J.H., Brollier, C., Bauer, D., & Schmidt, W. The Assessment of Occupation Functioning: The Second Revision. In J.H. Watts & C. Brollier (Eds.), *Instrument development in occupational therapy* (pp. 61–88). New York: Haworth, **1989.**

Watts, J.H., Kielhofner, G., Bauer, D.F., Gregory, M.D., & Valentine, D.B. (1986). The Assessment of Occupational Functioning: A screening tool for use in long-term care. *American Journal of Occupational Therapy, 40*(4), 231–240.

COST: ¢

SAMPLE:

Do you believe you make good use of your time? Give an example. (Values)
Do you feel in control of your life? For example, do you make your own decisions? (Personal causation)

❑ Canadian Occupational Performance Measure, Second Edition (COPM)

AUTHORS: Mary Law, PhD, OT(C), Sue Baptiste, MHSc, OT(C), Anne Carswell, PhD, OT(C), Mary Ann McColl, PhD, OT(C), Helene Polatajko, PhD, OT(C), and Nancy Pollock, MSc, OT(C)

FORMAT: Interview-based rating scale.

PURPOSE: This individualized client-centered outcome measure was designed to detect change in a client's self-perception of occupational performance over time. It is used to identify problem areas in occupational performance, evaluate client perceptions of performance and satisfaction with that performance, and measure changes in these perceptions. Thus the client is included in the treatment planning process.

POPULATION: Clients with a variety of disabilities and across all developmental stages (successfully used with children as young as 7 years). (Pilot testing included 256 clients at 55 sites in Canada and elsewhere.)

SETTING OR POSITION: Not prescribed.

MATERIALS OR TOOLS: Manual, rating cards, score sheet, and a pencil.

METHOD: Based on the Model of Occupational Performance (see Manual), the instrument is divided into three subareas: self-care, productivity, and leisure. Using unstructured interview, the therapist asks the client to report on occupational performance (describe the occupations he or she normally does), identifying problems in occupational performance and rating them in terms of importance (from 1= not important at all, to 10 = extremely important). The client then selects up to 5 problems that are most important and rates them in terms of performance (from 1 = not able to do it at all, to 10 = able to do it extremely well) and satisfaction (1 = not satisfied at all, to 10 = extremely satisfied). For clients with cognitive impairments, family or caregivers may respond. COPM yields total scores for performance and satisfaction. As an outcome measure, it should be administered at the beginning of occupational therapy and at intervals thereafter. Administration time is typically 30–40 minutes.

INTERPRETATION: The scores are used to compare clients' self-perceptions against their own reassessment scores; changes of 2 points are clinically significant. The problem list generated by the client forms the basis of intervention goals. Total scores can be used for program evaluation.

RELIABILITY: Test–retest reliability within a 2-week interval for 27 senior citizens receiving physical rehabilitation services was .63 for performance and .84 for satisfaction, using interclass correlation coefficients. A similar study with children is in progress.

VALIDITY: Validity was determined by examining how responsive COPM scores are to changes in self-perceived occupational performance over time. This was demonstrated by statistically significant differences in performance and satisfaction scores on reassessment, differences in outpatient scores after rehabilitation over a 3-month interval, and correlation of score changes with functional changes perceived by caregivers and others. COPM scores correlated more highly with independent ratings of client function than did two other occupational performance measures studied.

SOURCE: Available from: Canadian Association of Occupational Therapists, 110 Eglinton Avenue West, 3rd Floor, Toronto, Ontario M4R 1A3 Canada; 416-487-5404; Fax 416-487-0480. (**1991, revised 1994**)

COST: $

SAMPLE: **Productivity**
Paid/Unpaid Work (e.g., finding/keeping a job, volunteering)
Household Management (e.g., cleaning, laundry, cooking)

❑ Comprehensive Occupational Therapy Evaluation (COTE)

AUTHORS: Sara J. Brayman, MS, OTR, Thomas Kirby, PhD, Aletha M. Misenheimer, COTA, and M. J. Short, MD

FORMAT: Behavioral rating scale.

PURPOSE: The COTE was developed to provide a standard and objective method of observing and rating behaviors of psychiatric patients on a regular basis. It can serve as an initial evaluation and progress record to assist with treatment and discharge planning.

POPULATION: Adult acute psychiatric patients. (Sample consisted of community psychiatric hospital patients in a South Carolina hospital.)

SETTING OR POSITION: OT clinic; activities are suggested for observing behaviors.

MATERIALS OR TOOLS: COTE Scale and Definitions; pencil.

METHOD: The scale identifies 25 behaviors as observable in occupational therapy. These are divided into three areas: General Behavior, Interpersonal Behaviors, and Task Behaviors. The behaviors are rated by the therapist on a scale of 0 (normal) to 4 (greatest impairment), based on criteria listed for each item. The therapist rates the client on all behaviors at each session, providing a simple record in which the individual's behaviors can be compared over time. Each recording requires 2 minutes.

INTERPRETATION: COTE yields a daily summary of the client's behavior over the entire acute care hospitalization.

RELIABILITY: Interrater reliability is good (.95 average) for ratings within one degree of each other.

VALIDITY: Scores obtained on first day of hospitalization were compared with predischarge scores, and significant improvements in ratings were noted on the latter.

SOURCES: Brayman, S. J., & Kirby, T. (1976). Comprehensive Occupational Therapy Evaluation. *American Journal of Occupational Therapy, 30*(2), 94–100.

Brayman, S. J., & Kirby, T. Comprehensive Occupational Therapy Evaluation. In B. Hemphill (Ed.), *The evaluation process in psychiatric occupational therapy.* Thorofare, NJ: Slack, **1982.**

COST: ¢

SAMPLE:

General Behavior: Responsibility. (Ratings range from:)
0—takes responsibility for own actions [to]
4—denial of all responsibility; messes up project and blames therapist or others

❒ Functional Performance Record (FPR)

AUTHOR: David Mulhall

FORMAT: Observation-based checklist and database.

PURPOSE: This clinical instrument is intended for recording the observable actions and behaviors of people whose physical, social, or psychological functioning is impaired. It is used to identify the subject's assets and needs, set goals, evaluate the effectiveness of treatment, and assist with placement decisions. While the FPR serves as a record of the individual's level of function, the *Database* software can monitor standards of care, program planning, and research on a wide-scale basis.

POPULATION: Anyone with functional problems, including those with physical disabilities, learning disabilities, long-standing psychiatric disabilities, children in the care of social services, and more. (Research sample is not described.)

SETTING OR POSITION: Not specified. It is assumed that observations take place in the subject's environment.

MATERIALS OR TOOLS: Handbook and record form, pencil, and *FPR Database*.

METHOD: There are three components to the FPR: Checklist of over 600 items in 27 areas of function; *FPR Database* for transferring individual client information as well as storing multiple records; and the Handbook, which describes the use, administration, interpretation, and development of the FPR. The 27 topics cover a wide range of function, such as domestic/survival skills, aggression, feeding, socially unacceptable behavior, and speech and language reception. Each topic is arranged hierarchically, so that the broad topic includes defined questions containing specific items. The Checklist questions ask how the subject behaved during the last week. They are completed by the examiner after a week's observation of the subject or discussion with caregivers. Responses are recorded in response boxes according to various response options given for each question (e.g., degree of independence, frequency of behavior). Three columns of response boxes allow for retesting. Each of the topics is self-contained and can be used independently, so the evaluator can cover only relevant material for a wide variety of subjects.

INTERPRETATION: Each topic page stands alone as a summary of function in that area. The Handbook contains Training Notes to suggest intervention strategies based on topic results. The *Database* can produce statistical and graphical analysis of the descriptive information. The printouts provide convenient summaries and allow for easy comparisons of behavior. The *Database* also computes the "percentage support need" (i.e., degree of dependence) in the form of a bar graph. The FPR has been used by health authorities as a computerized register or central database for a particular population.

RELIABILITY: Interrater reliability was determined by two examiners of 12 residents in a psychiatric hostel. The percentage of agreement on choice of topics for all subjects was .80, agreement on the percentage support need ratings was .85 or above , and agreement on item responses was .70–1.00.

VALIDITY: Face and content validity are evident in the development and piloting of the questionnaire for a day center for people with physical disabilities. The questions and responses were refined by a wide variety of experts to improve clarity, objectivity, and range. There are no statistics on this.

SOURCE: Published by: NFER-NELSON Publishing

Company Ltd., Darville House, 2 Oxford Road East,
Windsor, Berkshire SL4 1DF England. Tel. (0753)
858961; Fax (0753) 856830. **(1989)**

COST: $$; Software $$$

SAMPLE: Hearing

What hearing difficulties did s/he have during the last week?

	with aids	without aids
In places with little background noise:		
responding when called by name	_ _ _	_ _ _
following one-to-one conversations	_ _ _	_ _ _
Responding to:		
telephone bells	_ _ _	_ _ _
doorbells/knockers	_ _ _	_ _ _

❑ Occupational Case Analysis Interview and Rating Scale (OCAIRS)

AUTHORS: Kathy L. Kaplan, PhD, OTR/L and Gary Kielhofner, DrPh, OTR, FAOTA

FORMAT: Semi-structured interview and rating scale.

PURPOSE: Based on the case analysis method for the model of human occupation, the OCAIRS provides a structure for gathering, analyzing, and reporting comprehensive data on the extent and nature of the subject's occupational adaptation. It is designed for discharge planning as well as eliciting self-evaluation, treatment planning, and community adjustment on the part of the patient.

POPULATION: Short-term psychiatric inpatients who show sufficiently organized behavior to participate in an interview. (Sample consisted of nine depressed or schizophrenic patients, ages 19–60.)

SETTING OR POSITION: Not prescribed; there should be no interruptions.

MATERIALS OR TOOLS: OCAIRS information, interview, rating, and summary forms and a pencil; audio- or videotape, if desired and permitted. An audiotape of case samples is provided for training the interviewer.

METHOD: The interview consists of 39 guided questions in 11 areas from the model of human occupation (e.g., values, interests, roles, habits). The manual provides guidelines for conducting the interview and adapting it to the individual. The interviewer takes notes on the responses and, following the interview, evaluates the material using a 5-point ordinal (rank-ordered) scale, according to specific descriptors for each rank. In addition to these 11 ratings, 4 global ratings are made about the subject's functioning as determined by system analysis: dynamic assessment (current functioning), historical assessment (past functioning), contextual assessment (environmental influence), and system trajectory assessment (direction of change). The 14 ratings and related comments are recorded on the summary form. Administration requires 20–35 minutes, with 30–50 minutes to score, record, and interpret. The interviewer must be a skilled clinician familiar with the model of human occupation.

INTERPRETATION: The 14 ratings yield a profile of strengths and weaknesses as defined by the theoretical model. The descriptive data represent the subject's self-perception and self-report, which explain the reasoning behind the ratings.

RELIABILITY: Interrater reliability on the research version was determined by four raters using intraclass correlation coefficients and ranging from high (.81–1.0) to fair (.21–.4) on the individual component ratings. The revised version was tested on 4 subjects with fewer high reliability ratings; small sample size may have affected results.

VALIDITY: Content validity was determined by a panel of 15 experts in the theory and psychosocial clinical practice areas; revisions were based on their input. Domain validity was confirmed by 15 therapists who matched interview questions to components of the model (82–100% correct, except habits 75% and output 70%). Concurrent validity studies compared OCAIRS with the Assessment of Occupational Functioning (high correlation) and with the Global Assessment Scale (moderate).

SOURCE: Published by: Slack Incorporated, 6900 Grove Road, Thorofare, NJ 08086. Tel: 800-257-8290; Fax: 800-853-5991. (**1989**)

COST: $

SAMPLE:

When people ask you what you do, what do you tell them?...

Rating

5   Realistically describes many (five or more) activities or obligations of a primary role. ...

3   Realistically describes one or two activities or obligations of a primary role. ...

1   Does not describe a primary role.

❑ Occupational Performance History Interview (OPHI)

AUTHORS: Gary Kielhofner, DrPH, OTR, FAOTA, Alexis D. Henry, MS, OTR/L, and Deborah Whalens, OTR/L

FORMAT: Semi-structured interview.

PURPOSE: OPHI is designed to gather a history of the individual's work, play, and self-care performance based on the Model of Human Occupation. It offers a view of how the subject perceives his or her life as well as the degree of adaptiveness exhibited.

POPULATION: Adolescents and adults, whether psychiatric or physically disabled, with adequate communication and attention. (Reliability study consisted of 4 groups totalling 154 clients in the following areas: adolescent psychiatry, adult psychiatry, physical disabilities, and gerontology.)

SETTING OR POSITION: Not prescribed.

MATERIALS OR TOOLS: Manual, interview form (a version based on the Model or an alternate Eclectic version), and a pencil.

METHOD: The interview consists of 39 recommended questions covering five content areas of occupational performance: organization of daily routines, life roles, interests/values/goals, perceptions of ability and responsibility, and environmental influences. The interviewer structures the interview and identifies with the subject the "turning point" that divides the history into past and present. The interview requires 45–60 minutes, after which the interviewer quantifies the information, rating 10 items (2 for each content area) on a 5-point scale indicating the degree of adaptive occupational function.

INTERPRETATION: The OPHI yields a Life History Narrative (a summary of the qualitative data collected) and a Life History Pattern (5-item scale reflecting the degree of adaptiveness exhibited by the subject and the influence of the environment).

RELIABILITY: Test–retest reliability of videotaped interview and subsequent live interview 5–12 days later ranged from .55–.68 for past ratings and .31–.49 for present ratings; a discussion of the ratings is included. Past and present item–total correlations for the individual subscale ranged from .63–.91, indicating a homogeneous scale and subscale. A generalizability study (Kielhofner et al., 1991) determined that interviewers using different frames of reference (MOHO and eclectic) used the OPHI with moderate stability.

VALIDITY: Not discussed. Face and content validity are evident.

SOURCES: Published by: The American Occupational Therapy Association, Inc., 4720 Montgomery Lane, PO Box 31220, Bethesda, MD 20824-1220. Tel: 301-652-2682; Fax: 301-652-7711. (**1989**)

Kielhofner, G. (1995). *A model of human occupation: theory and application (second edition)*. Baltimore: Williams & Wilkins.

Kielhofner, G., Henry, A., Whalens, D., & Rogers, E.S. (1991). A generalizability study of the Occupational Performance History Interview. *Occupational Therapy Journal of Research*, 11, 292–306.

COST: ¢

SAMPLE: ENVIRONMENTAL INFLUENCES

Recommended Questions:
Who are the important people in your life?
What are the things where you (live, work, go to school, etc., as appropriate) that help you get along?

❐ Occupational Questionnaire

AUTHORS: Nancy Riopel, MS, OTR and Gary Kielhofner, DrPH, OTR

FORMAT: Self-report (written) or interview.

PURPOSE: This tool is designed to collect data on a patient's use of time in daily activities and how it relates to the patient's volition (values, interests, and personal causation).

POPULATION: Any adolescents or adults. (Sample consisted of 60 subjects, ages 65–99 years, from a senior center and a nursing home.)

SETTING OR POSITION: Not prescribed.

MATERIALS OR TOOLS: Questionnaire and pencil.

METHOD: From memory of a typical weekday and weekend day, subjects report their main activity for every half hour time slot during the day. All activities are listed, whether the activity is work, daily living task, recreation, or rest; each is then rated on the activity's interest and value to the subject and how well he or she does it.

INTERPRETATION: The instrument yields a configuration activity; percent of time in work, play, etc.; percent of activities having value, interest, and a sense of competence; and activities that contribute most to these dimensions.

RELIABILITY: Test–retest reliability with 2-week interval indicated .68 agreement on the specified activities and .87 agreement on type of activity, .77 for personal causation, .81 for values, and .77 for interests.

VALIDITY: Concurrent validity indicated correlations with the Household Work Study Diary: .82 on typical activities, .90 and .97 on leisure and work classifications respectively, and .84–.92 on feelings toward others.

SOURCES: Obtain from: Model of Human Occupation Clearinghouse, University of Illinois at Chicago, Department of Occupational Therapy (M/C 811), College of Associated Health Professions, 1919 West Taylor Street, Chicago, IL 60612-7250. Tel: 312-996-6901; Fax: 312-413-0256.

Smith, N.R., Kielhofner, G., & Watts, J.H. (1986). The relationships between volition, activity pattern, and life satisfaction in the elderly. *American Journal of Occupational Therapy, 40*(4), 278–283.

COST: ¢

SAMPLE: For me, this activity is: extremely important, important, take it or leave it, rather not do it; waste of time.

☐ Self Assessment of Occupational Functioning (SAOF) and Children's Self Assessment of Occupational Functioning

AUTHORS: Kathi Baron, MS, OTR/L, and Clare Curtin, MEd, OTR/L

FORMAT: Checklist.

PURPOSE: The SAOF and corresponding Children's SAOF provide a method for collaborative treatment planning between patient and therapist, based on the Model of Human Occupation (MOHO). The subject assesses his or her level of function, identifies strengths, and prioritizes areas for improvement.

POPULATION: Children, adolescents, and adults who seek occupational therapy services in any area of practice: SAOF for ages 14–85 years, Children's SAOF for ages 10–13 years; subject must have sufficient cognitive skills.

SETTING OR POSITION: Not prescribed; the administrator is advised to set up an appropriate environment and time.

MATERIALS OR TOOLS: Manual that includes an overview of the MOHO, instruction sheet, rating forms, Definition page, Treatment Plan page, and pencil.

METHOD: SAOF consists of a series of statements that are categorized according to the three subsystems of the Model of Human Occupation (volition, habituation, and performance). Each statement is a component function of the subsystem and is rated by the subject as a strength, adequate, or an area needing improvement. Priorities are then chosen from the latter and listed. Following a discussion of the treatment priorities, the Treatment Plan is completed in the subject's own words. The checklist can be self-administered, or the therapist may read the statements and record responses. Two versions have been developed for adults: Short (23 areas of function with a definition page for clarification) for higher level subjects, and Long (more guidance and

structure) for lower level subjects or for self-administration. The children's version contains 44 items in 5 categories. SAOF should follow other performance evaluations or interviews in the assessment process.

INTERPRETATION: The SAOF yields a treatment program that is meaningful to the therapist and client, with Goals and Plan of Action enumerated.

RELIABILITY: Not discussed except for consideration of the appropriateness, and hence reliability, of the subject.

VALIDITY: Content validity is based on literature review and surveys of MOHO experts who confirmed the theoretical basis and structural organization of the checklist as well as its clinical application.

SOURCE: Distributed by: Model of Human Occupation Clearinghouse, University of Illinois at Chicago, Department of Occupational Therapy (M/C 811), College of Associated Health Professions, 1919 West Taylor Street, Chicago, IL 60612-7250. Tel: 312-996-6901; Fax: 312-413-0256. (**1986** [**revised 1990**])

COST: $

SAMPLE: Values
> Doing activities that give me a sense of purpose.
> Having future goals.
> Having realistic expectations of myself.

Activities of Daily Living

and

Home Management

Assessments

❑ Arnadottir OT-ADL Neurobehavioral Evaluation (A-ONE)

AUTHORS: Gudron Arnadottir, MA, BMROT

FORMAT: Performance-based rating scale and check-lists.

PURPOSE: Based on the occupational performance frame of reference, this clinical assessment identifies neurobehavioral deficits, how they interfere with functional performance in activities of daily living, and how they relate to the location of cortical lesions. It is designed to assist therapists in clinical reasoning and decision making regarding treatment methods, prognoses, and levels of independence.

POPULATION: Patients over age 16 with neurobehavioral dysfunction of cortical origin. (A-ONE was prepared for a pilot study of 65 subjects. A normative sample of 79 nonneurologic patients from four hospitals in Iceland represented a cross-section of the population of Iceland.)

SETTING OR POSITION: A-ONE should be administered in the morning at the patient's bedside with a sink nearby, in keeping with the daily routine. The area is set up for the observation in advance, with all necessities within reach.

MATERIALS OR TOOLS: A-ONE Parts I and II, ADL items for dressing, eating, and grooming. Subjects should use their own clothes and toiletries, and any aids needed, including glasses, dentures, walking aids, etc.

METHOD: A-ONE consists of two parts. Part I includes the *Functional Independence Scale* and the *Neurobehavioral Impairment Scale*. The Neurobehavioral Impairment Scale contains two subscales to assess specific and pervasive neurobehavioral impairments (e.g., apraxia, spatial neglect); the author provides corresponding checklists with behavioral examples of each impairment. Part II transfers the impairment scores to a *Neurobehavioral Scale Summary Sheet*, which identifies the frequency of observed central nervous system (CNS) dysfunctions.

Prior to the evaluation, the examiner records indications of cognitive, communication, and perceptual impairments on the Neurobehavioral Pervasive Impairment Scale. ADL performance is observed in five functional domains: dressing, grooming and hygiene, transfers and mobility, feeding, and communication. During or following the observation, the Functional Independence Scale and the Neurobehavioral Specific Impairment Subscale are scored for level of independence in each component skill (IP score) and for type and severity of each neurobehavioral dysfunction item (NB score). Ideally, scores should be based on two or three ADL observations. The IP scores range from 0 (unable; totally dependent) to 4 (independent), and NB scores from 0 (no deficits observed) to 4 (unable to perform due to CNS dysfunction); scores on the two scales should be inversely related. Interpretation and scoring of Part I requires 25 minutes or less; therapists must be experienced and trained in CNS dysfunction and ADL evaluation to allow the necessary flexibility to the standard protocol. The author's book provides theory and guidelines, but training is recommended for the examiner.

INTERPRETATION: Functional Independence Scale domain scores indicate level of independence and assistance needed in each performance area, while neurobehavioral impairment scores identify deficits and their severity across the domains. The Neurobehavioral Scale Summary Sheet shows the frequency of each dysfunction component for planning treatment. This score indicates the level at which the patient should be approached in treatment. The neurobehavioral impairments may be located in the author's table of CNS lesions in order to localize the dysfunction to specific cortical lobes and possible subcortical areas, and to set more precise treatment goals.

RELIABILITY: A test–retest reliability study indicated all three scales were stable over two testings within 1 week, yet are capable of detecting change over a 3-week interval. Interrater reliability was established for Parts I and II: In a study of 20 patients, each rated simultaneously by two raters, the average agreement on all scales of Part I was .84, with statistically significant agreement on all but five items; average agreement on Part II was .76, with localization on six lobes surpassing the .70 base agreement level. Attendance at a training seminar is required of examiners for reliable administration.

VALIDITY: Content validity was provided by literature review in CNS dysfunction, neurobehavioral theory, and principles of occupational therapy, as well as by consultation with experts in occupational therapy and neurology. A normative study of 79 patients (see Population) indicated that performance expectations for normal adults would yield a perfect independence score and 0 on all neurobehavioral subscales. A concurrent validity study comparing average performance of a normative sample compared to a sample of 50 cerebrovascular (CVA) patients demonstrated that A-ONE differentiates between the two groups in both IP and NP scores. A second concurrent validity study compared results of neuroimaging with A-ONE scores yielding modest agreement. Item analysis exhibited strong correlations for most items on the functional scale; items within domains correlated better than items across domains; correlations of functional items to neurobehavioral items ranged from .18–.78 agreement.

SOURCE: Arnadottir, G. *The brain and behavior: Assessing cortical dysfunction through activities of daily living.* Philadelphia: Mosby. (**1990**)

COST: $; this does not include the training and certification workshops that are available.

SAMPLE: Dressing	IP Score	Comments and Reasoning
Shirt (or dress)	4 3 2 1 0	
Pants	4 3 2 1 0	

NB Impairment	NB Score	
Motor apraxia	0 1 2 3 4	
Ideational apraxia	0 1 2 3 4	

❏ Assessment of Motor and Process Skills (AMPS)

AUTHOR: Anne G. Fisher, ScD, OTR/L, FAOTA

FORMAT: Observation-based performance evaluation and rating scale

PURPOSE: AMPS provides an objective assessment of motor and process (organizational/adaptive) skills in the context of performing several familiar functional tasks of the subject's choice. It examines the relation between these skills and domestic, or *instrumental*, ADL (IADL) performance, identifies the underlying causes of IADL limitations for treatment planning, and predicts performance capability in other areas of IADL.

POPULATION: Children from age 5 years through older adults with developmental, psychosocial, neurological, or musculoskeletal conditions that impose functional limitations on IADL. AMPS is contraindicated for subjects who are unwilling or have no need to perform IADL.

SETTING OR POSITION: Distraction-free familiar environment where tasks would normally be performed, or a clinical setting simulating the usual environment.

MATERIALS OR TOOLS: Manual, including scoresheet, pencil, and a computer with the AMPS computer scoring program. All tools and materials needed for the selected task as described in the manual should be in their usual locations in the actual environment, or placed where the client would normally store them in the simulated environment.

METHOD: The test consists of 56 household tasks that vary in difficulty from the simple to the complex. Task requirements are described for each. Two or three familiar but challenging tasks are selected for the therapist to complete, each requiring 10 to 20 minutes. Administration and scoring take 30 to 60 minutes and involve: an interview to determine appropriateness of client and selected tasks; negotiation of a "task contract" describing conditions of the task; setting up of the environment; contract review; administration of assessment (administrator records observations); scoring and interpretation of results. The administrator rates 16 motor and 20 process skills on a scale of 4 (Competent) to 1 (Deficit), according to how each skill contributes to successful task completion. For the severely delayed or impaired client, training in the selected task may precede testing, and AMPS is used to assess ability after learning.

INTERPRETATION: The AMPS computer scoring program generates the following reports: client's strengths and weaknesses as observed across all tasks, raw scores on skill items for each task, and overall motor and process ability measures. The latter represents the ability of the subject and can be used to predict the subject's capability in other domestic tasks; it also provides a basis for measuring change and effectiveness of intervention. AMPS is criterion-referenced, with performance being compared to the standard of competence.

RELIABILITY: Test–retest and interrater and intrarater (single rater scores compared to expected scores) studies on multiple versions of AMPS are summarized and support high reliability. Revisions of earlier versions include clarifications of skill item definitions and scoring criteria to improve reliability. Internal consistency for tasks and items are ≥ .90.

VALIDITY: Factor analysis confirms two unidimensional constructs of motor and process domains. Correlations of items and tasks indicate that the tasks and items are universal and measure common constructs. Concurrent validity studies compare AMPS with Scales of Independent Behavior, Mini-Mental State Exam, Older Americans Resources and Services (OARS)

ADL and IADL scales, and the Functional Independence Measure. Performance on one task predicts performance on a second, indicating stability within a single session (motor .95, process .93) and stability between sessions (motor .93, process .80). AMPS ability measures were found to discriminate between disability and well samples, between different levels of independent living, and between contrasting age samples. Over 5000 North American, Scandinavian, and United Kingdom subjects and all 56 tasks have been entered into the AMPS database with evidence of cross-cultural and cross-gender universality of items and tasks.

SOURCE: Anne G. Fisher, ScD, OTR/L, FAOTA, AMPS

Project, Occupational Therapy Building, Colorado State University, Fort Collins, CO 80523. Tel: 303-491-6253. (**1990 [revised 1994]**)

Users must be trained in a 5-day AMPS training and calibration workshop. For information, contact Dr. Fisher.

COST: $$$ (Cost of the workshop includes manual and computer program.)

SAMPLE: Temporal Organization

Initiates—starts or begins doing an action or step without hesitation; implies an end to decision making.

❐ Barthel Index

AUTHORS: Florence I. Mahoney, MD, and Dorothea W. Barthel, BA, PT

FORMAT: Performance index based on observation, interview, or records.

PURPOSE: This simple index of independence reflects the functional status of hospital patients in activities of daily living and assesses change.

POPULATION: Designed for patients with neuromuscular or musculoskeletal disorders, it has been widely used with many diagnoses in the adult population.

SETTING OR POSITION: Not prescribed.

MATERIALS OR TOOLS: Index and pencil. Any aids or materials for performing activities of daily living will be necessary.

METHOD: The original Index consists of 10 items of self-care and mobility. It is simple enough to be used by anyone observing or familiar with the subject's performance. Each item is scored in intervals of 5 based on the amount of time and assistance required to perform the activity. Scoring criteria are provided for each item. Environmental conditions such as architectural barriers may affect the score. Total score ranges from 0 to 100, with items weighted by prioritizing the most critical activities (continence and mobility). Granger and Greer (1976) expanded the original instrument to improve its sensitivity by including 15 items rated on a 4-point scale and weighting the items to reflect the impact of the resulting deficit. Shah and colleagues (1989) modified it by increasing the number of score categories to improve sensitivity to change.

INTERPRETATION: The total score yields categories of functioning: intact, limited, helper, and null. Item scores are more significant than the total as they indicate where the deficiencies are. Total score of 100 indicates treatment should not be necessary. (See Validity for other score interpretations.) The Index should be administered at intervals before and during treatment in order to note progress. Lack of improvement as reflected by unchanging scores indicates poor potential for rehabilitation.

RELIABILITY: Interrater and test–retest reliability (.89) are reported high. Internal consistency was reported by Shah et al. (1989) to improve from .87 for the original instrument to .90 for rehabilitation commencement and .93 for discharge in the revised version. Item ranks differ significantly among populations of different countries.

VALIDITY: Validity studies were summarized by Jacelon (1986), indicating that the Barthel Index scores agree with other independent measures of physical disability, and also compare favorably with the content and scores of other ADL assessments. Subjects with scores > 60 are more likely to be discharged home, and between 21–60 have equal probability of discharge to home, rehabilitation, or long-term care facility. The Index has been found to be an accurate measure of ability, predicting outcomes of rehabilitation and progress during recovery. Barthel Index admission score for stroke patients was a better predictor of outcome than lesion size or location determined by computerized tomography. Factor analysis shows a high degree of communality to each item.

SOURCES: Mahoney, F.I., & Barthel, D.W. Functional evaluation: The Barthel Index. *Maryland State Medical Journal, 14,* 61–65. (**1965**)

See also: Granger C.V., & Barthel, D.W. (1976). Functional status measurement and medical outcomes. *Archives of Physical Medicine and Rehabilitation, 57,* 103–109.

Jacelon, C.S. (1986). The Barthel Index and other indices of functional ability. *Rehabilitation Nursing,* 2(4): 9–11.

Shah, S., & Cooper, B. (1993). Commentary on "A Critical Evaluation of the Barthel Index." *British Journal of Occupational Therapy,* 56(2): 70–72.

Shah, S., Vanclay, F., & Cooper, B. (1989). Improving the sensitivity of the Barthel Index for stroke rehabilitation. *Journal of Clinical Epidemiology,* 42: 703–709.

COST: ¢

SAMPLE:

	With Help	Independent
Feeding (if food needs to be cut up = help)	5	10
Bathing self	5	10

❏ Dysphagia Evaluation Protocol

AUTHORS: Wendy Avery-Smith, MS, OTR, Abbey Brod Rosen, MS, OTR, and Donna M. Dellarosa, OTR

FORMAT: Checklist based on observation and performance.

PURPOSE: This clinical evaluation of dysphagia is designed to provide an objective and reliable measure of swallowing function. It can be used to identify patients who require radiographic assessment, for examination of oral and pharyngeal impairments, and to determine treatment needs, as well as assist in staff training.

POPULATION: Adults with a wide variety of diagnoses that may be associated with acute or chronic dysphagia. (Reliability studies included 37 patients, ages 18–95 years, referred for dysphagia evaluation at The New York Hospital.)

SETTING OR POSITION: Proper positioning of the subject and standard hand position used by the therapist are described in the instructions.

MATERIALS OR TOOLS: Manual of Dysphagia Assessment and Intervention, evaluation form, administration flipbook, and a pencil. Additional common test items are needed: flashlight, tongue depressor, stethoscope, spoon, adapted feeding devices as needed, surgical gloves, and food samples from five consistency categories (moist cohesive, soft chewable, thick liquid, thin liquid, and crunchy chewable).

METHOD: The evaluation form is divided into 11 sections: 5 history and status areas (feeding history, nutritional status, respiratory status, general observations, and physical status) and 6 clinical evaluation areas (observations, oral control, pharyngeal control, and feeding trial with oral stage and pharyngeal stage). The history and status are ascertained from direct and indirect sources: patient records, staff, caregivers, and questioning and observation of the subject. The clinical evaluation involves observation of oral characteristics, testing of oral–pharyngeal movements, sensation, and reflexes, and a feeding trial. The instructions include precautions, symptoms of aspiration, and contraindications for initiating or continuing the evaluation. (The manual also includes sections on alternative administration for confused patients, videofluoroscopic evaluation, tracheostomy and pulmonary considerations, pathology of the esophagus, dysphagia treatment techniques, and diet and nutrition.)

INTERPRETATION: The evaluation yields a summary of findings, a functional level indicating the degree of assistance needed, and recommendations for diet, therapy, or additional referrals. The recommendations provide a program plan, indicating treatment and feeding plans and precautions as well as any need for further consultation. Short- and long-term goals for therapy are developed from these recommendations.

RELIABILITY: Interrater reliability between pairs of occupational therapists ranged from 1.00–.85 with a median of .99 for two raters experienced with dysphagia, and 1.00–.90 with a median of .97 for experienced/inexperienced rater pairs. Test–retest reliability with 2-day intervals for inpatients and 1-week intervals for outpatients ranged from 1.00–.83 with a median of .93. (All correlations were based on raw scores.)

VALIDITY: Face and content validity are based on extensive literature review and collaboration with experts in dysphagia. Studies comparing videofluoroscopy with evaluation results are in progress.

SOURCE: Published by: Therapy Skill Builders, a division of Psychological Corporation, 555 Academic Court, San Antonio, TX 78204-2498. Tel: 800-228-0752; Fax: 800-232-1223. (**pending 1996**)

COST: $$

SAMPLE:

Pharyngeal Control:	Intact	Impaired	Absent	Comments
Soft Palate Function:				
Vocal Quality:				
Gag Reflex:				
Cough: volitional:				

❑ Elemental Driving Simulator (EDS) and Driving Assessment System (DAS)

AUTHORS: Rosamond Giatnutsos, PhD, Amy Campbell, OTR/L, Aaron Beattie, BA, and Frank Mandriota, PhD

FORMAT: Standardized computer-based performance simulation.

PURPOSE: EDS and DAS were developed to assess cognitive abilities necessary for safe driving and to demonstrate them to the subject sufficiently to promote correct decisions on whether and how to continue driving. These off-the-road assessments offer risk-free feedback to the subject and others on complex driving capabilities.

POPULATION: Cognitively at-risk drivers (e.g., older drivers, persons recovering from head injury or stroke). (DAS norms are based on 110 drivers without neurological diagnoses and ranging in age. EDS normative sample consists of 100 neurologically normal drivers ages 18–80.)

SETTING OR POSITION: Subject is seated in a chair in front of the driving console. Standard model steering wheel has adjustable position, and tension can be adjusted to the subject's motor abilities. The foot pedal assembly may be placed on the lap for hand operation. The examiner is seated at the computer.

MATERIALS OR TOOLS: Hardware that operates with an IBM or compatible computer consists of a steering console with a pedal floor plate and switch that accesses the personal computer (hemiplegia adaptive finger- and foot-switches available); computer software for task presentation and analysis; handbook and normative data. Additional programs for vision screening (REACT, SDSST, SEARCH, and SOSH) can be purchased. Portable or standard models are available.

METHOD: Determination of subject's eligibility should include screening of vision, motor function, and neurological status. The protocol begins with background information (including driving history) and a self-appraisal by the subject who rates on a continuum (worst—average) current cognitive abilities related to driving: reaction time, simultaneous processing, impulse control, ability to sustain performance, flexibility, eye–hand coordination, and judgment. Then each of the abilities is assessed in three (EDS) or four (DAS) increasingly complex simulated driving tasks. After the initial steering task, symbols are introduced to the EDS screen to which the subject must react in prescribed ways. EDS calculates six task measurements in addition to comparing response times across the three task phases. The DAS, however, proceeds from the initial task to increasingly complex pedal tasks in reaction to symbols on the screen. DAS summarizes eight performance measures with reaction time. EDS, the primary system, requires about 20 minutes, while the original DAS requires about 1 hour for a longer test protocol.

INTERPRETATION: The program prints two reports, the technical report and the personal report (printed in simple language for the subject). Both include norm-based score summaries, with performance ratings compared to self-appraisal ratings. This comparison tells whether subjects judge their own driving skills accurately, and by implication whether the individual is capable of exhibiting good judgment about driving. Cutoff scores are established, below which safe driving is rated unlikely. Simulation results suggest recommendations for further testing, training, or vehicle modifications (e.g., hand controls).

RELIABILITY: Internal consistency is reported high for performance ratings, as well as among subtasks (particularly those measuring the same skill), and for rank order of skill levels. Standard error confidence intervals are calculated for the EDS measures.

VALIDITY: Preliminary validation findings on EDS indicated consistent and substantial differences between older drivers and the normative sample; EDS produced a small but significant correlation (.08) with at-fault accidents. In a clinical rehab setting, statistically significant and clinically meaningful differences in on-road driving corresponded with EDS performance. (Note: EDS laterality index has proven to be a very sensitive measure of unilateral visual inattention [hemianopsia/ neglect]). Factor analysis identified five aspects of cognitive functioning measured by DAS and directly relevant to driving requirements. Predictive and concurrent studies are summarized comparing DAS with other procedures for driving advisement in rehabilitation settings, and comparing assessment results with driving practices 1 year later. Patients who failed overall clinical assessment also performed reliably worse on DAS measures, while patients who passed performed significantly better but not quite as well as the normative group.

COST: $$$$, includes software, hardware, mandatory training, seminar, and warranties; available only to those with professional credentials, such as OTR and COTA.

SOURCE: Materials and training available from: Life Sciences Associates, One Fenimore Road, Bayport, NY 11795-2115. Tel: 516-472-2111; Fax: 516-472-8146. **(DAS, 1992; EDS, 1994)**

❑ Evaluation of Oral Function in Feeding

AUTHOR: Margaret Stratton, OTR

FORMAT: Observation-based rating scale.

PURPOSE: The evaluation is designed to provide a uniform scale of oral function, based on objective and graded measures. It may be used to assess function over time, indicate need for intervention, or document function of client groups for comparison.

POPULATION: Multiply handicapped, developmentally disabled individuals. (Sample for reliability studies consisted of 46 severely and profoundly retarded, developmentally delayed residents of a state facility, ages 10 months to 21 years, who were dependent in feeding.)

SETTING OR POSITION: Not prescribed; subject should be in usual position for average meal.

MATERIALS OR TOOLS: Evaluation form, routine eating materials.

METHOD: The evaluation consists of nine feeding and related behaviors, including oral and facial movement and control, chewing, drinking, and swallowing. Each function is rated on a scale of 0 (passive) to 5 (normal), with written descriptions or criteria for each rating. In addition, positioning devices, reflex patterns, type of utensils, and diet should be noted. During an actual feeding session, the rater documents the level at which the subject eats without intervention or external controls by the feeder, if possible.

INTERPRETATION: The instrument yields a profile of oral function, with specific areas of strength or weakness noted.

RELIABILITY: Interrater reliabilities for two samples were .72 and .76; test–retest reliabilities were .68 and .79. Both are considered marginally acceptable by researchers, according to the author.

VALIDITY: Not reported.

SOURCES: Published in: Stratton, M. Behavioral assessment scale of oral functions in feeding. *American Journal of Occupational Therapy, 35*(11), 719–721. (**1981**)

Ottenbacher, K., et al. (1985). Reliability of the behavioral assessment scale of oral functions in feeding. *American Journal of Occupational Therapy, 39*(7), 436–440.

COST: ¢

SAMPLE: Lip closure over spoon.

(ranges from) 0: mouth remains open; no noticeable movement response to utensil.

(to) 5: lips purse together to actively remove food from bowl of spoon.

❏ Functional Assessment Scale (FAS)

AUTHOR: Estelle Breines, MS, OTR, FAOTA

FORMAT: Checklist-type rating scale.

PURPOSE: This scale is designed to provide a uniform, simple method of rating the level of self-care function/dysfunction in institutionalized patients. It is intended for clinical use, as well as research in monitoring an individual's progress or comparing groups of patients. Because it reflects only outcome performance, it should not be used as a sole clinical assessment.

POPULATION: Any hospitalized or otherwise institutionalized patient. (Research study sample included 249 patients in New Jersey nursing homes.)

SETTING OR POSITION: Not prescribed.

MATERIALS OR TOOLS: Functional Assessment Scale and pencil.

METHOD: The scale ranges from Level 1: "Total care" to Level 10: "Prepared to live independently." In between, the levels are defined by several functional capabilities, with criteria for each found in the manual. The rater checks each item the patient has mastered and scores according to the highest level in which the patient has mastered all items. The author recommends reevaluation every 2 weeks. Presumably the scale could be completed in several minutes by a rater familiar with the patient or by an observer.

INTERPRETATION: The scale yields a single level of function assigned to the patient. As an outcome measure, it monitors change without indicating underlying basis.

RELIABILITY: Interrater reliability is .95 per level, and .93 per item. The rater is encouraged to use clinical judgment in scoring.

VALIDITY: Content validity is based on review by a panel of experts and resulting field tests. FAS was found to accurately measure progress and decline in nursing home patients over time. Research is ongoing.

SOURCES: Published by: Geri-Rehab, Inc., 15 Hibbler Road, Lebanon, NJ 08833. Tel: 908-735-8918. (**1983**)

Breines, E. (1988). The Functional Assessment Scale as an instrument for measuring changes in levels of function for nursing home residents following occupational therapy. *Canadian Journal of Occupational Therapy,* 55(3): 135–140.

COST: $

SAMPLE: Level 6: Pushes wheelchair to destination. Follows safety precautions. Uses call system appropriately.

❑ Functional Behavior Profile (FBP)

AUTHORS: Carolyn Baum, MA, OTR/C, FAOTA, Dorothy F. Edwards, PhD, and Nancy Morrow-Howell, PhD, ACSW

FORMAT: Rating scale in checklist or interview format.

PURPOSE: The FBP provides caregivers with a method of describing the impaired person's *capabilities* in performing tasks, interacting with others, and solving problems. It is designed to assist in treatment planning, documenting change, and identifying helpful community resources.

POPULATION: Individuals with senile dementia of the Alzheimer's type (SDAT). (Sample consisted of 106 older adults living in the community with a caregiver.)

SETTING OR POSITION: Not prescribed.

MATERIALS OR TOOLS: Checklist and pencil.

METHOD: The FBP consists of 27 items relating to performance of daily activities by the cognitively impaired subject. The items are divided into three areas: task performance, social interaction, and problem solving. Each item is rated from 0 (never) to 4 (always), based on the subject's behavior over the past week. The checklist may be completed by the therapist by interviewing the primary caregiver, or by the caregiver independently. Administration requires 15 minutes. The FBP yields three scores: task performance factor, problem-solving factor, and social interaction factor. An institutional version of the Profile is available for residents of facilities.

INTERPRETATION: Lower scores indicate poorer performance. The authors suggest using the three scales independently to guide treatment, and they offer some intervention strategies.

RELIABILITY: Not discussed. The authors state the FBP should accurately reflect the caregiver's perceptions of the subject's capabilities in the three areas.

VALIDITY: The FBP was developed with input from families of SDAT patients. Factor analysis supported the creation of the three composite scales from the 27 items. Internal consistency of items is demonstrated for performance of tasks (.96), socialization (.94), and problem solving (.95). The three scales correlate with Short Portable Mental Status Questionnaire, Katz ADL Index, Zarit Memory and Behavior Problem Checklist, and Blessed Dementia Scale. Five problem-solving items were found to differentiate between the questionable and mild stages of the disease.

SOURCES: Obtain profile from: Carolyn Baum, MA, OTR/C, FAOTA, Washington University, 4567 Scott Avenue, St. Louis, MO 63105.

Baum, M.C., Edwards, D.F., & Morrow-Howell, N. (1993). Identification and measurement of productive behaviors in senile dementia of the Alzheimer type. *The Gerontologist*, 33(3): 403–408.

COST: ¢

SAMPLE: Finishes the tasks that have been started.

14_____13_____12_____11_____10

Always	Usually	Sometimes	Rarely	Never
(100%)	(80%)	(50%)	(20%)	(<10%)

❑ Functional Independence Measure (FIMˢᵐ) and Functional Independence Measure for Children (WeeFIMˢᵐ)

AUTHOR: Prepared by The Center for Functional Assessment Research at State University of New York at Buffalo, under the direction of Carl V. Granger, MD.

FORMAT: Rating scales based on observation of performance.

PURPOSE: The Uniform Data System for Medical Rehabilitation (UDSMR) is a nonprofit organization that promotes uniform documentation of the severity of patient disability and the results of medical rehabilitation. At the core of the UDSMR is the Uniform Data Set, which includes FIM and WeeFIM for assessing severity of disability. They are used as measures of functional status and reflect the impact of disability on the individual and on the human and economic resources of the community. FIM and WeeFIM are designed for clinical evaluation of the individual and to generate group data and analyze the outcomes of rehabilitation.

POPULATION: FIM is designed for adults, WeeFIM for children ages 6 months to 7 years. There are two versions of WeeFIM: inpatient for use in pediatric facilities; and community/outpatient for use in outpatient, school-based, and home-care settings.

SETTING OR POSITION: Not specified. The subject should perform the task as usual, in the setting most often used.

MATERIALS OR TOOLS: Guide, Coding Sheets, pencil, FIMware (software to document and track assessment results using Microsoft Windows). Other materials for performance of daily living tasks are used as needed.

METHOD: FIM and WeeFIM are interdisciplinary evaluations administered at designated time periods after admission and discharge from rehabilitation, long-term-care facilities, and in home care. Both instruments contain a 7-level scale that indicates major gradations from dependence to independence in activities of daily living and the degree of assistance required. Each consists of 18 areas of function scored from 1 (total assistance) to 7 (complete independence), according to written performance criteria for each item. Ratings are assigned by a clinician who observes the subject (FIM and WeeFIM) or who interviews the caregiver (WeeFIM). The subject must complete the stated tasks to qualify for a given level. Users of the instruments are encouraged to adopt additional items for their own clinical use if desired. The instruments yield total scores ranging from 18–126 as well as 2 domain scores (motor and cognitive), 6 subscale scores (self-care, sphincter control, transfers, locomotion, communication, and social cognition), and 18 individual item scores. Demographic and medical information is recorded if the examiner subscribes to the UDSMR database, an international accumulation of over one half million patient records.

INTERPRETATION: FIM and WeeFIM are measures of disability, not impairment. That is, the results reflect what the subject actually does, not is capable of doing. FIMware produces the FIM Profile that graphically displays current functional status and changes over time, gives norms or national median scores for comparison, and allows users to maintain their own database.

RELIABILITY: Interrater reliability was determined by pairs of clinicians from 89 U.S. rehabilitation facilities who evaluated 1,018 patients; intraclass correlation coefficients were calculated for total (.96), domain (motor .96 and cognitive .91), and subscale (.89–.94) scores (Hamilton, Laughlin, Fiedler, & Granger, 1994). To improve reliability, users may be trained by USDMR. Before their data may be entered into the USDMR database, users must be credentialed by USDMR with rater reliability above .80.

VALIDITY: A panel of interdisciplinary experts in pediatric rehabilitation rated the content validity of the WeeFIM (McCabe & Granger, 1990): they agreed on the assignment of domain and subdomain items, but not that the items adequately represented the subdomains. Research is ongoing. FIM scores were found useful in predicting burden of care as measured in minutes of physical assistance required per day, and they contributed to predictions of the level of subjects' satisfaction with life (Granger, Cotter, Hamilton, Fiedler, & Hens, 1990; Granger, Cotter, Hamilton, & Fiedler, 1993).

SOURCES: For information about AdultFIM (Version 4.0—1993), contact Jan Bailey. For information about WeeFIM (Version 4.0—1993), contact Susan Braun. Write to: Uniform Data System for Medical Rehabilitation, 232 Parker Hall, State University of New York at Buffalo, 3435 Main Street, Buffalo, NY 14214. Tel: 716-829-2076; FAX: 716-829-2080; e-mail: FIMNET@ubvms.cc.edu.

Granger, C.V., Cotter, A.C., Hamilton, B.B., & Fiedler, R.C. (1993). Functional assessment scales: a study of persons after stroke. *Archives of Physical Medicine Rehabilitation, 73*: 133–138.

Granger, C.V., Cotter, A.C., Hamilton, B.B., Fiedler, R.C., & Hens, M.M. (1990). Functional assessment scales: a study of persons with multiple sclerosis. *Archives of Physical Medicine Rehabilitation, 71*: 870–875.

Hamilton, B.L., Laughlin, J.A., Fiedler, R.C., & Granger, C.V. (1994). Interrater reliability of the 7-level Functional Independence Measure (FIM). *Scandinavian Journal of Rehabilitation Medicine, 26*: 115–116.

McCabe, M.A., & Granger, C.V. (1990). Content validity of a pediatric Functional Independence Measure. *Applied Nursing Research, 3*(3): 120–122.

COST: Guide—$$. On-site training—$$$$.

SAMPLE: BATHING Includes bathing (washing, rinsing and drying) the body from the neck down (excluding the back); may be either tub, shower or sponge/bed bath.

<u>NO HELPER</u>

7 Complete Independence—The child bathes (washes, rinses and dries) the body. Performs safely.

<u>HELPER</u>

1 Total Assistance—The child performs little or none (less than 25%) of bathing tasks.

❑ Geriatric Rating Scale/Stockton Geriatric Rating Scale

AUTHORS: R. Plutchick, PhD; H. Conte, MA; M. Lieberman, MS; M. Baker, MA; J. Grossman, PhD; and N. Lehrman, PhD (Geriatric Rating Scale); B. Meer and J. A. Baker (Stockton Geriatric Rating Scale)

FORMAT: Observation-based behavioral rating scale.

PURPOSE: The scale is designed to assess all behavior of patients that contributes to their being ready to leave the hospital as "improved." The Geriatric Rating Scale is a revision of the Stockton Scale.

POPULATION: Geriatric institutionalized patients, including those with functional psychotic disorders and organic mental disease.

SETTING OR POSITION: Not prescribed.

MATERIALS OR TOOLS: Rating scale and pencil.

METHOD: The 33 items on the Stockton Scale cover four factors: physical disability, apathy, communication failure, and socially irritating behavior. The 28-item Geriatric Rating Scale updated, deleted, and added a number of items. Scores are based on observations of behavior in self care, use of time, assistance needed, and interpersonal behavior. Nursing staff or attendants can rate a patient on a well-defined 3-point scale in 10 minutes.

INTERPRETATION: Each scale yields a total summed score, with higher scores indicating greater impairment. The Stockton Scale yields factor scores on individual skills.

RELIABILITY: Interrater reliability is reported to be .87 for both scales, and test–retest reliability over a 1-year interval is .65 for the Geriatric Rating Scale. Internal consistency of factors is demonstrated by factor analysis (ranging from .77 to .94 for Stockton, and .75 to .90 for Geriatric Rating Scale).

VALIDITY: Good predictive and discriminative validity is demonstrated. Stockton scores correlated with leaving the hospital, staying, or death and with improvement following electroshock therapy. Geriatric Scale discriminated between geriatric and nongeriatric patients, organic and functional psychotic patients, and with psychiatrist ratings.

SOURCES: Published in: Plutchik, R., Conte, H., Lieberman, M., Baker, M., Grossman, J., & Lehrman, N. (1970). Reliability and validity of a scale for assessing the functioning of geriatric patients. *Journal of the Geriatrics Society, 18,* 491-500.

Meer, B., & Baker, J.A. The Stockton Geriatric Rating Scale. *Journal of Gerontology, 21,* 392–403. (**1966**)

COST: ¢

SAMPLE: The patient will begin conversations with others:

> Often
> Sometimes
> Almost never

□ Katz Index of ADL

AUTHORS: S. Katz, A. B. Ford, R. W. Moskowitz, B. A. Jackson, M. W. Jaffe

FORMAT: Interview and observation.

PURPOSE: This index provides a relatively quick and easy ADL assessment, indicating level of independence/dependence and a general indication of the type of assistance required. Because of its general nature, it may be more useful as a research measure for change in status than as a clinical skills assessment.

POPULATION: Developed for use with the elderly and chronically ill. (Over 2,000 evaluations were administered to a sample of 1,001 individuals in good health or with a variety of diagnoses.)

SETTING OR POSITION: Not prescribed; may be dictated by activity assessed.

MATERIALS OR TOOLS: Evaluation form, pencil; additional materials as needed during ADL observation.

METHOD: The index assesses performance in six functions: bathing, dressing, using the toilet, continence, transferring, and eating. After questioning the subject or observing the performance in question, the examiner rates the subject as independent, assisted, or dependent.

INTERPRETATION: The data yield a grade from A (independent in all areas) to G (dependent in all 6 functions), indicating degree and general types of assistance needed.

RELIABILITY: Good interrater reliability is referred to by Katz, Downs, Cash, and Grotz (1963).

VALIDITY: Face, construct, and concurrent validity reported: Correlates with self concept of patients, discriminates between amount of attendant care required, and identifies sequence of improvements in patients. Predictive validity demonstrates .50 correlation with patient mobility, .38 with house confinement.

SOURCES: Katz, S., Ford, A.B., Moskowitz, R.W., Jackson, B.A., & Jaffe, M.W. The Index of ADL: A standardized measure of biological and psychosocial function. *Journal of the American Medical Association, 185*, 914–919. (**1963**)

Katz, S., Downs, T.D., Cash, H.R., & Grotz, R.C. (1970). Progress in development of index of ADL. *Gerontologist, 10*, 20–30.

COST: ¢

SAMPLE: Feeding:

Feeds self without assistance.	Feeds self except for getting assistance in cutting meat or buttering bread.	Receives assistance in feeding or is fed partly or completely by using tubes or intravenous fluids.

□ Kitchen Task Assessment (KTA)

AUTHORS: Carolyn Baum, MA, OTR/L, FAOTA, and Dorothy F. Edwards, PhD

FORMAT: Standardized performance-based rating scale.

PURPOSE: The KTA is designed as a practical and objective measure of organizational, planning, and judgment skills as performed in a common task. It provides information on the level of assistance necessary to support such performance, as well as recording change in the subject's function.

POPULATION: Adults with Senile Dementia of the Alzheimer's Type (SDAT). (Sample was 106 men and women, ages 53–84, with questionable to severe dementia, and living in the community with a caregiver.)

SETTING OR POSITION: Kitchen: counter, refrigerator, stove, and sink are used.

MATERIALS OR TOOLS: Setup of pudding mix, milk, saucepan, kitchen utensils, dishes, soap and paper towels is described. Instructions are printed on paper in large letters.

METHOD: A qualifying pretest of washing hands precedes the assessment to determine a minimum level of ability. The subject is then instructed and observed while making a cooked pudding from a mix. The administrator provides the assistance necessary for a successful experience. A score of 0 (independent), 1 (verbal assistance), 2 (physical assistance), or 3 (totally incapable) is given in six categories: initiation, organization, performing all steps, proper sequence, judgment and safety, and completion. The task takes about 15 minutes.

INTERPRETATION: The final score ranges from 0 to 18; the higher the score, the more impaired the performance. As a clinical tool, the performance on the subtests provides information and strategies useful to the caregiver.

RELIABILITY: Interrater reliability is .853 for the total score, ranging from .632 (safety) to 1.0 (initiation). Factor analysis yielded loadings exceeding .88, indicating high relationships among variables. High correlation coefficients (.72–.84) suggest that the domains measured all contribute to the cognitive dimension.

VALIDITY: Analysis of variance found KTA to discriminate among the different stages of the disease regardless of subject's gender. Construct validity is demonstrated by correlation of KTA with other neuropsychological and functional tests.

SOURCE: Baum, C., & Edwards, D. Cognitive performance in senile dementia of the Alzheimer's type: The Kitchen Task Assessment. *American Journal of Occupational Therapy, 47,* 431–436. (**1993**)

COST: ¢

SAMPLE: Performance of all steps: Did he or she perform all the major steps—measuring steps: stirring, pouring—alone? Did you have to assist him or her, for example, in lighting the stove? Was it verbal or physical assistance?

❏ Klein-Bell Activities of Daily Living Scale

AUTHORS: Ronald M. Klein, PhD, and Beverly J. Bell, OTR

FORMAT: Behavior rating scale.

PURPOSE: This scale is designed to provide a "reliable, quantitative and meaningful measure of independence in activities of daily living (ADL)" to be universally applicable. It is used to determine current level of functioning, follow progress, communicate to professionals and family, and allow specific and comprehensive treatment planning. It is appropriate for clinical purposes and research.

POPULATION: Intended for use with patient populations, ages 6 months to adulthood. (Studies completed on adult hospital patients and on 20 normal children and children with cerebral palsy, ages 13 months to 6 years.)

SETTING OR POSITION: Appropriate setting for observing the test behaviors; appropriate positions are stated for each area of testing, generally standing, sitting (including wheelchair), or lying.

MATERIALS OR TOOLS: Manual includes the ADL scale and scoresheet.

METHOD: The scale consists of 170 items in six areas of function: dressing, elimination, mobility, bathing/hygiene, eating, and emergency telephone communication. Each area is broken into subareas (e.g., eating solid food, semisolid food, etc.), which are further broken down into essential behavioral components. Each component is observed and scored: able to perform activity (i.e., independently), unable, or not applicable. Scores are weighted from 1 to 3 points for each component.

INTERPRETATION: Raw scores are obtained for each area and added together for a total score; percentage scores are indicated on the scoresheet. The test yields a profile of scores in the areas assessed.

RELIABILITY: Interrater reliability is .92 for raters inexperienced with the scale. In the children's sample, interrater and test–retest reliability were .99 and .98 respectively.

VALIDITY: Content validity is suggested by developing a scoring system based on numerical ratings by experts. Preliminary studies of predictive validity indicate a correlation (-.86) between discharge scores and number of hours of daily assistance required at home 5 to 10 months later. Construct validity is supported by the ability of baseline scores to differentiate between normal children and children with cerebral palsy, and by agreement of scores with parental ratings of performance.

SOURCES: Obtain from: Health Sciences Center for Educational Resources, University of Washington, T-281 Health Sciences Building, Box 357161, Seattle, WA 98195-7161. Tel: 206-685-1186 (Distribution); Fax: 206-543-8051. **(1982)**

Law, M., & Usher, P. (1988) Validation of the Klein-Bell Activities of Daily Living Scale for Children. *Canadian Journal of Occupational Therapy*, 55(2), 63–68.

COST: ¢; instructional video $$

SAMPLE: Comb hair
              Grasp comb/brush
              Comb top hair
              Comb back hair
              Release comb/brush

☐ Kohlman Evaluation of Living Skills (KELS), 3rd edition

AUTHORS: Linda Kohlman Thomson, MOT, OTR, OT(C), FAOTA

FORMAT: Interview and task performance tests.

PURPOSE: This tool is designed to provide a quick and simple evaluation of an individual's ability to perform basic living skills. Although not comprehensive, it can help determine degree of client's independence and suggest appropriate living situations that will maximize independence.

POPULATION: Created for short-term psychiatric adolescent and adult inpatients based on urban American culture, but wider application includes clients who are mentally retarded, geriatric, brain injured, or cognitively impaired. The assessment categories are not applicable to long-term care settings. (Several studies used samples of up to 50 patients.)

SETTING OR POSITION: Subject is seated to left of or across from evaluator.

MATERIALS OR TOOLS: Three-ring binder, test manual including test forms and scoresheet, and additional common materials (bar of soap, telephone book and telephone, pencil, deck of cards, $2 and change).

METHOD: The instrument includes 17 items in five categories: Self-Care, Safety and Health, Money Management, Transportation and Telephone, and Work and Leisure. The items comprise a sample of basic living and community skills. For each item, instructions, materials, and scoring criteria are prescribed. Each item is scored as independent (0) or needs assistance (1 1/2 or 1 point). Additional comments on client's test behavior are summarized on the scoresheet. Administration requires 30–45 minutes.

INTERPRETATION: The test yields a single cutoff score indicating capability to live independently in the community. The results are intended to be analyzed by the clinician in order to recommend appropriate training and disposition, based on the scoresheet profile.

RELIABILITY: Interrater reliability in an early study ranged from .74 to .94 agreement. Subsequent studies reported on by the author use minor changes in procedure and yield high agreement (.84, .94, .94, .98, 1.00).

VALIDITY: The author summarized concurrent validity studies that compared KELS with the Global Assessment Scale (.78–.89 agreement) and BaFPE (-.84; due to opposite scoring direction, this indicates high agreement), and found KELS scores to distinguish between clients in sheltered housing versus those living independently. Two unpublished predictive validity studies were summarized: KELS successfully predicted which of 20 geriatric clients could live successfully in the community; a second study of psychiatric clients showed wide variation of results possibly due to flawed research design.

SOURCE: American Occupational Therapy Association, Inc., 4720 Montgomery Lane, PO Box 31220, Bethesda, MD 20824-1220. Tel: 301-652-2682; Fax: 301-652-7711. (1992)

COST: $

SAMPLE: Safety and Health

1. Awareness of dangerous household situations (from photographs).
   I am going to show you four pictures. There may be a dangerous situation in them, or there may not be anything dangerous at all. Look carefully at each of them.

❏ Milwaukee Evaluation of Daily Living Skills (MEDLS)

AUTHOR: Carol A. Leonardelli

FORMAT: Observation-based rating scale, time limited.

PURPOSE: This behavioral assessment is intended to provide a standard, quantifiable measure of daily living skills for lower-functioning, long-term psychiatric clients. It is designed to be easy to use and sensitive to the effects of treatment and to aid in treatment planning and goal setting.

POPULATION: Adults, ages 18 and over, who are chronically mentally ill (at least 2-year history), including residents (at least 6 months' duration) of psychiatric facilities, skilled nursing facilities, halfway houses, and group homes, or participants in outpatient and day treatment programs (for at least 2 years). (Sample consisted of 26 adult males residing in a community facility in a small town in Wisconsin.)

SETTING OR POSITION: Generally not prescribed but may be inferred from item descriptions.

MATERIALS OR TOOLS: MEDLS manual, including screening and reporting forms; an equipment list is provided for each subtest, consisting primarily of common consumer items (e.g., ADL supplies).

METHOD: The evaluation consists of 20 subtests that are observed by the rater during actual or simulated performance of daily living skills. Standard instructions and a time limit are provided for each item. A skill list for each item breaks down the activity into component steps that make up the grading criteria. The rater scores each item from 0 (unable to perform any skills) to 4 (performs all skills). Scores are not cumulative; that is, the test yields a list of 20 item scores. The evaluation is administered individually and requires up to 2 hours, excluding eating time; it may be administered in more than one session. The evaluator may use the screening form to determine which areas to assess and which are not indicated, based on background or initial information.

INTERPRETATION: The test scores provide an indication of performance in daily living skills to be used as a baseline for treatment and to measure progress.

RELIABILITY: Interrater reliability ranges from .40 to 1.00 for 17 of the 20 subtests, with most at .80 or above.

VALIDITY: Content validity is demonstrated by literature review and consultation with experts. The author recommends that criterion-related studies be carried out.

SOURCE: Leonardelli, C.A. *The Milwaukee Evaluation of Daily Living Skills: Evaluation in long-term psychiatric care.* Thorofare, NJ: Slack. (**1988**)

COST: $

SAMPLE: Nail Care

<u>Skill List</u>
a. Trims fingernail neatly and safely
b. Trims toenail neatly and safely
c. Cleans nails (finger and toe)
d. Cleans up area

❏ Parachek Geriatric Rating Scale

AUTHOR: Joann Frazier Parachek, PhD

FORMAT: Observation-based behavior rating scale.

PURPOSE: This tool is intended to assist hospital and professional personnel in treatment planning for elderly patients, by grouping them according to ability and potential. It provides a simple and quick screening method for charting capabilities and changes of the most general nature and might best be used by support personnel. A treatment manual accompanies it.

POPULATION: Geriatric inpatients. (Sample consisted of 150 psychiatric patients over age 65 at Arizona State Hospital.)

SETTING OR POSITION: Not prescribed.

MATERIALS OR TOOLS: Parachek Geriatric Rating Scale and Treatment Manual.

METHOD: The patient is rated by the observer in three categories: physical capabilities, self-care skills, and social interaction skills. There are a total of 10 broadly defined items, which are rated by checking one of five descriptive statements most appropriate to the patient. These range from dependent to independent status and determine the item score. A caregiver familiar with the patient could complete the scale in a few minutes.

INTERPRETATION: The instrument yields a total score that allows the patient to be grouped according to three general levels of function described in the treatment manual. The manual describes the population falling in each range and makes treatment recommendations.

RELIABILITY: None reported.

VALIDITY: Criterion and concurrent validity reported: .88 with the Plutchik Geriatric Rating Scale; .77 with

initial diagnostic classification indicates it is effective for quick screening and to select patients for treatment programs.

SOURCES: Published by: Center for Neurodevelopmental Studies, 5430 West Glenn Drive, Glendale, AZ 85301. Tel: 602-915-0345. (**3rd edition, 1986**)

Miller, E.R., & Parachek, J.F. (1974). Validation and standardization of a goal-oriented, quick-screening geriatric scale. *Journal of the American Geriatrics Society*, *22*, 278–283.

COST: ¢

SAMPLE: Hygiene:

(ranges from) l. Must be bathed by aides . . .

(to) 5. Keeps self clean and bathes or washes by self.

❑ Performance Assessment of Self-Care Skills, version 3.1 (PASS)

AUTHORS: Joan C. Rogers, PhD, OTR/L, and Margo B. Holm, PhD, OTR/L

FORMAT: Observation-based performance rating.

PURPOSE: PASS is designed to provide data about daily living skill performance in the clinic or in the home. It establishes a baseline functional status, measures change at discharge, and assists in treatment and discharge planning by identifying the type and amount of assistance required for successful performance.

POPULATION: Adults in the occupational therapy clinic or in the home. (Administered to over 400 adults from healthy and from diagnostic populations such as arthritis, cardiopulmonary disease, dementia, depression, mental retardation, and schizophrenia.)

SETTING OR POSITION: Setup for each task is described in the rating protocol, for both clinic and home versions.

MATERIALS OR TOOLS: Kit includes manual, scoresheets, and standardized stimulus items. Additional common items for self-care performance are listed in the manual for purchase by the examiner. Authors recommend that the kit for the home version be transported in a small rolling suitcase.

METHOD: PASS consists of 26 tasks: 5 functional mobility (MOB), 3 personal self-care (ADL), and 18 instrumental activities of daily living (IADL). Two versions, PASS-Clinic and PASS-Home, accommodate to each environment. The PASS rating protocols describe the context (e.g., bathroom, bedroom), setup, and verbal instructions for each item. The items are subdivided into critical subtasks for rating purposes. This allows the examiner to identify the specific point or points in the task sequence where performance breaks down and to codify the type and number of task or context modifications or human assists necessary for safe and successful task completion. Items are scored on a 4-point ordinal scale. Since PASS is criterion-referenced (subject is rated according to established performance criteria), it may be given in total, or selected items may be used alone or in combination. Administration of all 26 items takes 1 1/2 to 3 hours to complete.

INTERPRETATION: PASS yields three types of summary scores: Independence on each subtask and Safety and Outcome for each of the 26 tasks. The three ratings identify task abilities and disabilities and determine whether disabilities are due to deficits in independence, safety, or quality of task outcome.

RELIABILITY: Interrater reliability of PASS-Clinic (version 2.0) based on 1,965 observations of 30 subjects by 2 observers yielded agreements on Performance Score (.96), Independence Score (.99), Person Assists (.99), and Task/Environment Assists (.99). The same agreements were reached by 2 observers for the PASS-Home (2.0). Agreements by 3 observers of 5 subjects in both settings ranged from .93–.99. Internal consistency of specific items on PASS ranged from .89–.93 for MOB and ADL Scales and .93–.95 for IADL. Interrater and test–retest reliability studies for PASS 3.1 are in progress.

VALIDITY: Content validity of PASS is based on investigation of ADL/IADL categories, tasks, and task specifications in several ADL and functional assessment tools used in geriatrics and rehabilitation. Construct validity is evident from two studies. In the first, IADL scores were proportionally lower and more variable than ADL scores in patients with primary degenerative dementia; in the second, performance scores were higher for control subjects than for patients with depression, and lowest for patients with dementia.

SOURCE: Publication pending. Information currently

available from the authors at: WPIC #1237, 3811 O'Hara Street, Pittsburgh, PA 15213.

COST: Kit expected to be $$.

SAMPLE: IADL: Medication Management

"Please read the prescription label and find the directions for taking this medication [hand patient bottle with child-proof lid and wait until patient looks up]. If you were taking this medication *today*, when would you have to take the next pill?" [Wait for response].

❑ Scorable Self-Care Evaluation (Revised)

AUTHORS: E. Nelson Clark, MS, OTR/L, and Mary Peters, MS, OTR

FORMAT: Standardized test based on observation, interview, and performance.

PURPOSE: This self-care evaluation instrument is designed to provide a comprehensive, quantifiable, and brief measure of functional performance and to identify problems in basic living skills. It can be used to obtain a baseline profile, communicate progress, plan treatment, and guide discharge plans.

POPULATION: Adolescents and adults; the instrument is designed to be appropriate for individuals with psychiatric disorders in acute and community settings. It does not yet consider the needs of the physically disabled. (Norms are based on a sample of 67 students and employed persons, all residing in the San Francisco area and ranging in age from 13 to 62 years.)

SETTING OR POSITION: Subject seated comfortably at a table 30 inches high, examiner seated directly across with manual and shield.

MATERIALS OR TOOLS: Manual and work/scoring sheets, pencils, local map, 16 3" x 5" cards as directed, telephone numbers, telephone directory, play money.

METHOD: The evaluation is composed of 18 subtasks, divided into four subscales: personal care, housekeeping chores, work and leisure, and financial management. Prior to each subscale, a Motivation Questionnaire is administered to determine the subject's beliefs and values toward self-care skills. Performance tasks and observations are then administered with standardized instructions and scoring criteria provided for each item. Points are assigned in each subtask for the inability to perform the task. Scores are tabulated to obtain subscale scores and a total score. Administration of the test ranges from 35 to 65 minutes. Recommended treatment tasks are offered for deficits revealed by the evaluation.

INTERPRETATION: Subscale scores are plotted on the data record to yield a profile of scores ranging from "functional" (top of graph) to "dysfunctional" (bottom of graph). Percentage scores are provided. Low scores are interpreted as requiring "skill development."

RELIABILITY: Test–retest reliability with a 2-month interval was reported good for all but the personal care subscale. Interrater reliability for total scores based on rating already completed responses ranges from 1.00 to .86. All subscale correlations are reported significant. Most item-to-subscale and item-to-total correlations are significant; all four subscales achieved strong correlations with the total score.

VALIDITY: Survey of the literature indicates content validity; further research is in progress, including a survey of occupational therapists.

SOURCE: Published by: Therapy Skill Builders, a division of Psychological Corporation, 555 Academic Court, San Antonio, TX 78204-2498. Tel: 800-228-0752; Fax: 800-232-1223. (**1984, revised 1993**)

COST: $

SAMPLE: First Aid Bleeding

State: How do you stop bleeding, such as a bad cut or nosebleed?

❏ Structured Observational Test of Function (SOTOF)

AUTHORS: Alison Laver, OTR, with Graham E. Powell

FORMAT: Observation and question-based performance test.

PURPOSE: SOTOF was developed to provide a detailed description of functional status and associated neuropsychological deficits within a structured evaluation of activities of daily living. It serves as a screening tool to describe individuals who need intervention, provides a baseline for treatment planning, and assists in diagnosis.

POPULATION: Older adults with possible neurological disturbance or dementia. (Normative speed and performance data are based on a sample of 86 adults, ages 60–97, without neurological diagnoses or deficits.)

SETTING OR POSITION: Any suitable clinical or home setting with minimal noise and distraction, good lighting, and comfortable temperature. Setup of materials is described for each task.

MATERIALS OR TOOLS: Manual, Instruction Card booklet, record forms, and pencil. In addition, a table, two chairs, and common ADL objects preferably belonging to the subject (unbreakable cup and bowl, nonslip mat, soap, food, any necessary assistive devices, etc.) must be assembled.

METHOD: SOTOF consists of five subtests with an Instruction Card for each: a Screening Assessment to identify level of functioning and eligibility for testing, and observation of four simple ADL tasks. The examiner observes the subject performing four personal daily living tasks (eating, washing, pouring and drinking, and dressing) and asks questions about the tasks. The Instruction Cards suggest possible deficits for each component step, and additional prompts or assessments to gain more information. The Screening Assessment is scored Able/Unable in each of five categories (vision,

sitting balance, etc.) with observations and hypotheses recorded. The ADL and Neuropsychological Record Form is scored by indicating on the score sheet whether the subject performs the task independently, what skills are intact (e.g., reaching, sequencing), what problems are evident (e.g., perceptual, motor), and what the underlying dysfunction (e.g., agnosia) might be. Guidelines are provided for scoring descriptive responses to test questions. SOTOF takes about 10–15 minutes for the normal sample to complete.

INTERPRETATION: SOTOF yields information on four levels of function: ADL performance, specific skills and deficits, performance components, and underlying neuropsychological deficits. Summary observations and hypotheses are written descriptively.

RELIABILITY: Internal consistency was established between ADL tasks and Neuropsychological Checklist; ADL task variability indicated all tasks must be administered to complete the assessment. The author reports high to acceptable levels of test–retest (1-day interval) and interrater reliability, respectively, at .92 (97.7% agreement) and .94 (97.5%) on Screening Assessment, .5–.77 (90.3–93.8% agreement) and .37–.67 (89.5–91.6%) on four ADL tasks, and .55 (95.2%) and .54 (95.2%) on Neuropsychological Checklist. A high degree of clinical judgment is inherent in the scoring, influencing these values (percentage agreement and Kappa statistics used).

VALIDITY: Face validity was demonstrated by clients who reported the tasks to be representative of typical activities. Content validation was provided by literature review and by surveys and interviews of experienced occupational therapists who helped define the constructs to be evaluated (perception, cognition, motor, and sensory function), the criteria for evaluation, and the task components by activity analysis. Construct and concurrent validity were further demonstrated by agreement between SOTOF and other ADL and neuropsychological tests in identifying ADL dysfunction and neuropsychological deficits. Therapists reported good clinical utility of the test (quick, easy, relevant to clients, etc.).

SOURCE: Published by: NFER-NELSON Publishing Company Ltd., Darville House, 2 Oxford Road East, Windsor, Berkshire SL4 1DF, England. Tel: (0753) 858961; Fax (0753) 856830. (**1995**)

COST: $$

SAMPLE: **Pouring and Drinking**
Ask: "What can you see on the table?"
Ask: "Which is the jug, mug, cup?"
Instruct: "Put the cup on the table on the left of the jug."
Ask: "What do you use these objects for?"

Vocational

Assessments

Adult Skills Evaluation Survey for Persons with Mental Retardation (ASES)

AUTHORS: Jane T. Herrick, OTR, and Helen E. Lowe, OTR

FORMAT: Performance-based rating scale.

PURPOSE: ASES was developed to fill a need for a vocational assessment for mentally retarded adults. It is used to assess skills associated with successful vocational performance and evaluate problem areas needing intervention. It is designed to define specific needs, set appropriate goals for vocational training, and measure progress and program accountability.

POPULATION: Adults with mild to moderate mental retardation. (Although the authors report using the ASES with several hundred clients of the Now Opportunity Workshops, Inc., no data are offered on the sample.)

SETTING OR POSITION: Private, quiet location without distractions. Subject is seated comfortably at a table with examiner seated in full view.

MATERIALS OR TOOLS: Manual and record sheets. The examiner needs to assemble a long list of common items and tools, including several that require simple construction (e.g., cardboard shapes, tool construction board), and that are stored according to authors' suggestions.

METHOD: ASES estimates performance in three domains: fine motor skills, perceptual skills (visual and auditory), and acquired skills. There are six to eight items in each section; for every task, the subject is rated on a 6-point scale according to written criteria (from 0–makes no attempt to..., to 5–performs...correctly). The evaluation yields subtest scores, section scores, and a total survey score. Observations on performance and personal characteristics are rated separately. It is administered individually and requires 1 to 2 hours. The examiner can pace the testing to the client's attention span and energy level.

INTERPRETATION: Test scores indicate potential for functioning in vocational training programs and in supported employment. Scores are plotted on the Individual Profile to present a composite picture of strengths and weaknesses. Performance is also charted on two graphs: the Prediction of Performance in a Work Setting (scores rated from good ability to no ability) and the Progress Graph.

RELIABILITY: Interrater reliability between the examiner and a co-rater scoring simultaneously was .58; as a result, the authors further refined the instructions and scoring procedures for the present edition. Research is ongoing.

VALIDITY: Content validity is supported by a survey of vocational training personnel who rated the importance of client success factors. The survey has not been analyzed statistically. Research is ongoing.

SOURCE: Obtain from: Helen E. Lowe, 770 North Fair Oaks Avenue, Pasadena, CA 91103. Tel: 818-449-0969; Fax 818-449-0994. **(1990, 3rd edition)**

COST: $

SAMPLE:	PERCEPTUAL SKILLS FOLLOW DIRECTIONS	
	Stand up.	I'M GOING TO TELL YOU 3 THINGS TO DO. (Hold up 3 fingers.) LISTEN TO ALL 3. (Point to your ear.) DO EXACTLY WHAT I SAY. ARE YOU READY?
	Place a chair elsewhere in the room.	STAND UP, PUSH YOUR CHAIR UP TO THE TABLE, AND GO SIT IN THAT CHAIR.

❐ APTICOM®

AUTHORS: Vocational Research Institute (VRI) division of the Philadelphia Jewish Employment and Vocational Services (JEVS)

FORMAT: Computerized battery of performance tests and questionnaire.

PURPOSE: APTICOM provides a quick criterion-referenced vocational assessment in three major areas: aptitudes, interests, and educational levels. It is most useful as an initial evaluation in schools, rehabilitation hospitals, community vocational programs, private industry, and correctional facilities to offer meaningful job recommendations. It was developed in part to reduce boredom and anxiety from longer vocational testing.

POPULATION: English- or Spanish-speaking disadvantaged job applicants, high school or special education students, and rehabilitation clients. (Norms are based on two nationwide samples: 856 prevocational secondary school students or subjects under 18 years, and 525 vocational postsecondary students over age 18 and adults in rehabilitation, job training, or other vocational counseling programs.)

SETTING OR POSITION: Computer requires tabletop at which subject is seated; height and dimensions are described in the manual.

MATERIALS OR TOOLS: The APTICOM system is a self-contained unit consisting of a dedicated microcomputer, several testing devices consisting of a plastic board (18" x 24") with an array of holes corresponding to test answers and plastic overlay panels for the different tests, a response wand, and various computer controlled devices for measuring dexterity aptitudes; a printer and paper are required.

METHOD: This self-timing and self-scoring computer-ized system consists of a Vocational Aptitude Battery, Educational Skills Development Battery, and Occupational Interest Inventory, with a Data Entry System for Report Customization. The system contains an administrative manual with directions and scoring instructions and a technical manual with development and interpretation sections for each part of the battery. All instructions are oral with some demonstration, and a practice trial is given before each test. Except for the Interest Inventory, the number of correct responses comprise raw scores. The computer will complete all scoring and explain the results in the final report.

The Vocational Aptitude Battery contains 11 subtests measuring 10 aptitudes (e.g., object identification, clerical matching, eye–hand coordination), each taking several minutes. Reading ability is required on only 2 subtests, which are written at the fourth grade reading level.

The Occupational Interest Inventory comprises 162 items, using an answer format of "like"-?-"dislike" and requiring 15–20 minutes to complete.

The Educational Skills Development Battery contains two 30-item tests, each requiring 10–15 minutes: Language Skills and Math Skills.

INTERPRETATION: The final report can be printed from the APTICOM computer or downloaded on a personal computer. The report contains raw and standard scores and percentiles for the aptitudes; raw and standard scores and percentiles of interest areas compared to the norms, with a statistical analysis of high interest areas; and math and language skills scores with a content analysis. Based on high interest areas and aptitude scores, vocational recommendations are made for all viable Work Groups (as defined by U.S. Department of Labor) with examples of specific jobs, and cross-classification of interest, aptitude, and educational levels.

RELIABILITY: Test–retest reliability of aptitudes range between .65–.89 (most above .80) with substantial standard error of measurement reported. Test–retest reliability of the 12 interest areas ranged from .74–.86 and compared favorably with the USES Interest Inventory.

VALIDITY: The aptitude and interest components of the APTICOM were validated against the Department of Labor General Aptitude Test Battery (GATB), a much longer test, with correlations of .81–.87 for the three cognitive aptitudes, .65–.67 for perceptual aptitudes, and .37 and .52 for dexterity skills. Factor analysis yielded three factors: cognitive, perceptual, and motor. Correla-

tions ranged from .72–.85 between the Interest Inventory and the widely used USES Interest Inventory scores. Content validity is demonstrated for the Educational Skills Development Battery by experts in vocational evaluation and language development who analyzed items according to U.S. D.O.L. General Educational Development (GED) definitions.

SOURCE: Obtain from: Vocational Research Institute, 1528 Walnut Street, Suite 1502, Philadelphia, PA 19102. Tel: 1-800-VRI-JEVS. (**1981, latest revision 1992**)

COST: $$$$+ (Several system options are available at a range of prices.) $$ for an optional training videotape with workbooks.

SAMPLE: Contact publisher.

◻ The Geist Picture Interest Inventory: Revised

AUTHORS: Harold Geist, PhD

FORMAT: Checklist using picture selection method.

PURPOSE: This inventory was developed to identify occupational choices and the motivation behind the choices. The use of pictures and drawings to illustrate the occupations is intended to decrease the ambiguity of verbal titles, offer a projective component for additional information, and to facilitate use among the verbally impaired and illiterate.

POPULATION: Norms are available by sex, age, education, and different ethnic, occupational, and psychopathological groups from 8th grade through adulthood. (Pilot sample consisted of 1,500 boys and girls grades 4 through 12 in four California communities.)

SETTING OR POSITION: Not prescribed.

MATERIALS OR TOOLS: Manual, Picture Triad Booklets for Male and Female, Motivation Questionnaires for Male and Female, and pencil.

METHOD: The Inventory is self-administered individually or in groups. The subject is given the appropriate Triad Booklet, which contains trios of drawings representing major vocations and avocations. (Male contains 132 drawings depicting 113 activities and 19 objects associated with activities; Female contains 81 drawings of 68 activities and 13 objects.) Only occupations common to the U.S. are included. Clarifying questions are written under each triad; these may be read to the subject. The subject circles the drawing of his or her choice within each trio. On completion, the Motivation Questionnaire may be completed by the subject identify-ing which of seven reasons influenced each choice (e.g., family, prestige, financial). The three strongest motivations are recorded. The interest areas are totalled and may be graphed on the Interest Profile.

INTERPRETATION: Totals are converted to normalized scores: over 70 indicates strong interest and under 30 indicates dislike. For each interest area identified (11 for males, 12 for females), descriptions are offered along with suggested jobs or occupations. Further exploration may be offered by the counselor. Each of the seven motivation areas is totalled and converted to percentages to estimate the relative strength of each motivating force. These may be graphed on profile summaries.

RELIABILITY: Reliability is increased by use of drawings over verbal stimuli according to the author and by pretesting the drawings for accuracy and ease of identity. Test–retest reliability over 6-month intervals is summarized for various male and female samples, indicating high levels of statistical significance in nearly all groups.

VALIDITY: Most correlations between 10 of the interest areas and 10 Kuder Scale interests reach statistical significance. Author indicates Geist scores are more valid than Kuder scores with subjects who have reading handicaps. Correlation with grades, parent ratings, and work satisfaction in 5-year follow-up studies also are stated to support the validity of the Geist with grades 8 through 12, college, and adult groups.

SOURCE: Published by: Western Psychological Services, 12031 Wilshire Boulevard, Los Angeles, CA 90025. Tel: 800-648-8857; Fax: 310-478-7838. (**1982**)

COST: $$

SAMPLE: Triad Drawings:

1. Chemist	Tree Surgeon	Radio Announcer
2. Actor	English Teacher	Music Conductor

❑ Jacobs Pre-Vocational Assessment (JPVA)

AUTHOR: Karen Jacobs, MS, OTR

FORMAT: Observation-based performance tasks.

PURPOSE: JPSA is designed to assess performance in specific work-related skill areas among adolescents with learning disabilities. It may be used as a screening tool for planning treatment and referrals.

POPULATION: Preadolescents and adolescents with learning disabilities. (Developed for this population at the Learning Prep School.)

SETTING OR POSITION: Not prescribed; generally subject is seated at table except for environmental mobility task.

MATERIALS OR TOOLS: Manual and Profile Sheet (both found in text referenced below); a list of common items and other materials that can be readily made or purchased. The author suggests organizing all material in a carrying case.

METHOD: The JPSA consists of 15 brief tasks (e.g., filing, factory work, money concepts) assessing 14 skill areas (coordination, cognition, and perceptual skills). Each task is described in the manual, including purpose, materials, and instructions; examples of task modifications are offered for special needs. Skill areas required by each task (4 physical capacities, 6 work behaviors, and 5 work aptitudes) are checked off on a checklist-style Profile Sheet. The therapist circles any areas of difficulty observed during the assessment and records the time needed to complete each task (up to the maximum time permitted). Scoring criteria are not offered, thus relying on therapist judgment. The test requires 1 to 2 hours, and yields a pattern of checks and circles on the Profile Sheet. In addition, the therapist notes any significant behaviors displayed during testing (e.g., hand domi-nance, cooperation, perseverance), as well as modifications or adaptive equipment needed.

INTERPRETATION: Any physical capacity, work behavior, or work aptitude with two or more circled checks on the Profile Sheet indicates areas for remediation in therapy. Sample evaluation reports are offered for summarizing and reporting results.

RELIABILITY: Not discussed.

VALIDITY: Author consulted other therapists and standardized instruments in developing this assessment, analyzing and categorizing tasks, and refining the revised version as a result of clinical use.

SOURCE: Jacobs, K. *Occupational therapy: Work-related programs and assessment, second edition.* Boston: Little, Brown. (1991)

COST: $$

SAMPLE: Money Concepts

"You are a sales clerk in a store, and I am a customer who would like to buy this magazine. Here is a dollar. ... Please give me the correct change."...

McCarron-Dial System (MDS) and Perceptual-Motor Assessment for Children (PMAC)

AUTHORS: Lawrence McCarron, PhD, and Jack G. Dial, PhD

FORMAT: Standardized norm-based battery of behavioral and psychometric measures.

PURPOSE: This comprehensive work evaluation system is designed to assess educational and vocational potential of the neuropsychologically disabled population in vocational, educational, and clinical settings. It is used to identify neuropsychological strengths and weaknesses and to assist in program planning.

POPULATION: Individuals with neuropsychological impairment, ages 16 years and above; a screening version for children ages 4 through 15 is also available. (Original sample consisted of 200 clients of rehabilitation settings, daycare, training, and employment programs; other studies include subjects who are blind, adults from ages 19–69 who are psychiatrically disabled, adults and children who are deaf, and subjects who are mentally retarded, spinal cord injured, closed head injured, or learning disabled.) General population norms are described in each manual.

SETTING OR POSITION: Described individually by the standardized test manuals comprising the battery.

MATERIALS OR TOOLS: Each standardized instrument with manual and materials is available from MDS, except for the Wechsler tests and the Peabody, which are used in interpreting the results but are not part of the battery. An instructional overview of the system is available from the publisher, as well as computer programs to assist in computing and interpreting data and writing reports.

METHOD: MDS is based on the measurement of three neuropsychological factors (verbal-spatial-cognitive, sensorimotor, and emotional-coping) and their ability to predict the vocational competency of the individual. Three methods of data gathering are used: history taking, behavioral observation, and standardized testing. An outline of topics, questions, and descriptions is provided for the first two methods.

Standardized testing uses: the Wechsler Adult Intelligence Scale–Revised or Wechsler Intelligence Scale for Children–Revised, the Peabody Picture Vocabulary Test–Revised, and the Bender Visual Motor Gestalt Test (for visual-motor integration scoring only, not projective interpretation).

In addition, MDS developed the following instruments for the battery: the Haptic Visual Discrimination Test, McCarron Assessment of Neuromuscular Development (MAND), Observational Emotional Inventory (involving 2 hours of observation of the subject each day for 5 days), Dial Behavior Rating Scale, and the Street Survival Skills Questionnaire (which may also be used as an independent measure). Other instruments are added or substituted depending on the nature of the evaluation, disability, setting, and age of subject.

Raw score distributions for each predictor and criterion variable are transformed to standard scores and represented graphically by the Individual Evaluation Profile and Individual Program Plan; computer programs may be purchased for computing and interpreting data and generating reports. Training in the MDS is needed.

Perceptual-Motor Assessment for Children (PMAC) is a 9-part multiple-choice screening version of the MDS for children that assesses verbal/cognitive/academic, sensory/motor, adaptive/coping, and emotional/behavior performance. (The 35-item emotional behavior questionnaire is optional.) PMAC requires 45 minutes to administer.

Modifications of the MDS are available for the blind/

visually impaired; an abbreviated version of the MDS (see Validity) does not use the Wechsler tests, which are restricted in use to specifically qualified personnel anyway.

INTERPRETATION: The Individual Evaluation Profile summarizes the subject's performance on the three factors and provides norms for comparison of scores to special and general populations, identification of individual strengths and deficits in the major factors, and predictions of vocational and residential program levels (five levels each and expected range of earnings); this helps in developing and prioritizing general program goals. The Individual Program Plan organizes the factor data to identify specific strengths and deficits for individual program planning.

PMAC yields: the Comprehensive Evaluation Report itemizing scores and profiling strengths and weaknesses, and the Classroom Report summarizing functional behaviors and assisting school staff in daily programming.

RELIABILITY: Extensive reliability (test–retest, interrater, and split-half) studies are summarized in the individual test manuals. Test–retest reliability coefficients range from .67 (in one subtest) to .99 for the MAND (fine = .98, gross = .96, total = .99) and .90 and .93 for the Haptic. Retesting the subject over a 1-month interval is suggested as an indication of the stability of performance scores over a short period.

VALIDITY: Studies of the neuropsychological factors to predict vocational competency over an 18-month interval yielded correlations of .90 to the vocational competency scale and .70 to the work sample. Factor analysis yielded the three neuropsychological factors. Extensive research documents content and construct validity; concurrent validity of MDS to rehabilitation

program placement and of an abbreviated battery to predicting vocational competency; predictive validity to program placement, wage earnings, and functional living levels (e.g., Haptic to work potential ranged .53–.86, MAND to work performance was .70); and the use of MDS data for program applications and treatment. Clinical studies demonstrate its use in identifying learning disabilities and in discriminating among various population combinations affected by brain lesions and brain damage, normal, psychiatric, and cerebral palsy.

SOURCES: Produced by: McCarron-Dial Systems, PO Box 45628, Dallas, TX 75245. Tel: 214-247-5945. (MDS 1973; last revised 1986) (PMAC 1988)

Chan F., Lynch, R.T., Dial, J.D., Wong, D.W., & Kates, D. (1993). Applications of The McCarron-Dial System in vocational evaluation: An overview of its operational framework and empirical findings. *Vocational Evaluation and Work Adjustment Bulletin, 26*(2), 57–65.

COST: $$$$[+] for MDS; $$$$ for PMAC; $$$–$$$$ for computer programs. $$$ for 3-day workshops and on-site training provided by MDS.

SAMPLE: Haptic Visual Discrimination Test—Familiarization

Instruct the subject: **"Place your right hand through this opening." ..."Look at each of these shapes pictured here...I am going to put a shape just like one of these in your hand...but you will not be able to see it."**...

❐ Reading-Free Vocational Interest Inventory

AUTHOR: Ralph L. Becker

FORMAT: Standardized forced-choice inventory, self-administered.

PURPOSE: The inventory is designed as a nonreading vocational preference test, based on pictorial illustrations, rather than verbal or written statements. It is intended for use with individuals having limited verbal or reading ability. Identifying areas and patterns of interest aids vocational counseling and job placement.

POPULATION: Adolescents and adults who are mentally retarded and learning disabled, age 13 and over. (Normative sample included educable students who are mentally retarded and learning disabled, grades 7 through 12 in public schools, and adults who are mentally retarded, ages 17 to 59, in sheltered workshops and vocational training centers, from geographic divisions representing all regions in the U.S.)

SETTING OR POSITION: Not prescribed.

MATERIALS OR TOOLS: Manual, inventory booklet with individual profile sheet, pencil.

METHOD: The inventory booklet contains 165 pictures of occupational activities appropriate to this population. Eleven interest areas are represented, such as automotive, clerical, animal care, housekeeping, and horticulture. The illustrations are arranged in sets of three, or triads, and the subject circles the preferred item in each triad. The inventory may be completed in 20 minutes or less and can be administered individually or in a group.

INTERPRETATION: The test yields a numerical score for each interest area that is converted to a percentile rank and charted on the profile sheet. The final graphic display identifies high, average, and low interest areas.

RELIABILITY: Test–retest reliability, over a 2-week interval for each norm category, is generally good (.70s and .80s). Internal consistency (median .82) indicates reliability of content.

VALIDITY: Content validity is based on the study and categorization of appropriate jobs and their depiction in clear line drawings. Concurrent validity is demonstrated by correlations with the Geist Picture Interest Inventory. The inventory is shown to discriminate among occupational groups.

SOURCE: Published by: Elbern Publishing, PO Box 09497, Columbus, OH 43209. Tel: 614-235-2643; Fax: 614-237-2637. (**revised, 1981**)

COST: $

SAMPLE: "There are many rows of pictures of people working at different jobs . . . be sure you circle one picture in each row."

❏ Valpar Component Work Sample Series and Dexterity Modules

AUTHORS: Varied, with the collective effort of the Valpar Corporation.

FORMAT: Standardized task performance simulating job activities.

PURPOSE: The Work Sample Series is designed to generate clinical and actuarial data on universal worker characteristics. Keyed to worker traits in the Dictionary of Occupational Titles (DOT), the series indicates the subject's ability to be a successful worker in the area(s) sampled as well as providing activities for therapy. The Dexterity Modules are intended to assess hand, upper extremity, and visual coordination functions.

POPULATION: Designed for use by disabled or nondisabled persons, there may be adaptations or restrictions for the visually impaired or blind. (Normative samples of nondisabled employed workers and special disability groups are available for most work samples.)

SETTING OR POSITION: Evaluation area should be well-lighted, clean, and relatively free of noise and visual distractions.

MATERIALS OR TOOLS: Each work sample consists of manual and standardized equipment ranging from common items (tape recorder) to large equipment especially designed for the work sample. Dexterity s consist of a base unit and pegboard-style apparatus. Stopwatch, pencil, and scoring sheet are required. Standard-size tables and chairs or stools may be needed.

METHOD: The Series consists of 23 Work Samples, each assessing groups of skills making up a type of employment task (such as mechanical or clerical), or specific components (such as ROM and eye-hand-foot coordination). Many of the samples are made up of several exercises that may be given individually, in combination, or in entirety. Entire samples range in time from 20–90 minutes to administer. All but the cooperative assembly task are administered individually. Samples may be administered repeatedly to improve performance. Each manual includes a list of materials, evaluator's preparations, standardized instructions to the client, timing and scoring directions, and a rating system for worker characteristics (e.g., ability to follow instructions, concentrate on tasks, communicate, make decisions). A separate kit contains tactile or verbal modifications to adapt Samples for the visually impaired. In addition, System 2000 consists of software to analyze the scores of three work samples, convert scores with other systems, produce work history, match subjects to jobs, and more.

Series 300 Dexterity Modules consist of 5 independent units administered singly as indicated. They are: small parts assembly, asymetrical pin placement, tool manipulation, bimanual coordination, and angled pin placement.

INTERPRETATION: Each work sample is described by a Worker Qualifications Profile (WQP), which analyzes the skills, factors, and work-related aptitudes required to complete the task successfully. Methods–Time Measurement (MTM) determines whether the subject meets an industry standard of speed and accuracy for completing the sample. Normative tables provide error and time percentile scores for each exercise (Valpar assists in developing local norms), however Valpar recommends evaluating scores based on work requirements and not just by comparison to others. Graduated scoring tables encourage repeated test administrations in order to learn the skill.

RELIABILITY: Samples 1 to 16 of the original series have test–retest reliability ranging from .70 to .99 for work rate and accuracy scores, based on samples of 50 subjects over 1-week intervals.

VALIDITY: The work samples have been criterion-referenced according to the domain of the Department of Labor's extensive job analysis and classification system (refer to the DOT and Revised Handbook for Analyzing Jobs). Furthermore, the work samples have been analyzed using MTM engineering to establish time rates representing standards of a well-trained worker. Valpar's face validity may improve worker motivation and appeal. (Dexterity Modules have recently been developed, and research was not reviewed in time for publication of this text.)

SOURCE: Valpar Corporation, 3801 East 34th Street, Suite 105, Tucson, AZ 85713. Tel: 800-528-7070; Fax: 520-292-9755. **(Work Samples: 1974, most manuals revised by 1994) (Dexterity Modules: 1995)**

COST: $$$$–$$$$[+]; $$$—each Dexterity Module

SAMPLE: General Clerical

Say: This is a work sample designed to see how well you can perform certain tasks that often are required of persons working in an office. The sample is divided into three sections: Telephone Answering, Mail Sorting, and Alphabetical Filing. I will show you how to do each of these tasks... .

☐ Vocational Interest, Temperament and Aptitude System (VITAS)

AUTHORS: Vocational Research Institute (VRI) division of the Philadelphia Jewish Employment and Vocational Services (JEVS)

FORMAT: Standardized work samples.

PURPOSE: VITAS uses realistic work simulation to assess vocational aptitudes, interests, and temperaments for vocational guidance and placement. In use by schools, job training programs, rehabilitation centers, and correctional centers, it was designed to provide comprehensive short-term evaluation of large numbers of clients.

POPULATION: Secondary school students and adults, ages 14 years and up. (Norms are based on 325 culturally/educationally disadvantaged adults and 225 special needs high school students.)

SETTING OR POSITION: Not prescribed.

MATERIALS OR TOOLS: Manual, behavior observation record and scoresheets, profile sheets and report forms (all forms available in English and Spanish), individually packaged work sample hardware (materials, tools, and equipment).

METHOD: VITAS in its entirety consists of 22 work samples, or for more limited assessment is divided into four clusters of 5–10 interrelated samples: Mechanical-Industrial I, Mechanical–Industrial II, Clerical–Business Detail, and Technology. In each work sample, the client performs a task that is identical or similar to a job experience, with actual materials used in work settings. While the client performs the work sample, the evaluator records observations on aptitudes and behavior. The sample is scored for time and quality of work. Following the completion of the samples, the evaluator meets with the client to complete the Vocational Interest Interview Form to elicit interests and review performance. Each of the clusters requires 3 to 4 1/2 hours to administer; the entire VITAS takes 2 1/2 days. (When the entire VITAS is being administered, a motivational group session follows the first day.) A 6th grade reading level is required.

INTERPRETATION: The Evaluation Report is a synthesis of the interest interview, recorded observations, and performance scores. It describes the client's appearance, attendance, and punctuality; verbal ability; interpersonal behavior; and skills and aptitudes. Recommendations for supportive services are made, and placement in work groups or training is based on norm comparisons (in accordance with the U.S. Department of Labor's Guide for Occupational Exploration, 1979, available from VRI).

RELIABILITY: Test–retest reliability is not studied, as the work samples are experiential methods that rely on learning effects; no alternate forms or equivalent devices are available.

VALIDITY: Face, content, and construct validity are summarized in an unpublished study submitted to the Department of Labor and unavailable to the public. The VITAS tasks were found to be representative of 16 Work Groups in the Guide for Occupational Exploration. Independent teams analyzed the samples for construct validity.

SOURCE: Obtain from: Vocational Research Institute, 1528 Walnut Street, Suite 1502, Philadelphia, PA 19102. Tel: 1-800-VRI-JEVS. **(1980)**

COST: $$$$⁺: for the basic system, expanded system, or cluster packages; includes training and certification (encouraged but not required for clusters). $ for supplementary resources, such as the Guide for Occupational Exploration or Dictionary of Occupational Titles.

SAMPLE: APTITUDES

Numerical: Ability to perform arithmetic operations quickly and accurately.
Clerical Perception: Ability to perceive pertinent detail in verbal or tabular material. ...

❏ Vocational Adaptation Rating Scales (VARS)

AUTHORS: Robert G. Malgady, PhD, and Peter R. Barcher, PhD

FORMAT: Standardized rating scale of typical behaviors.

PURPOSE: The VARS were developed to measure maladaptive behavior likely to occur in a vocational setting that might jeopardize the employment status of a mentally retarded worker. Information gained from VARS is intended to guide remediation efforts, assist with placement decisions, and supplement data for vocational evaluation.

POPULATION: Male and female adolescents and adults, ages 13 to 50, ranging from borderline to severely retarded. (Sample is 606 individuals who are mentally retarded, primarily young adults with mild to moderate retardation, in two New York counties.)

SETTING OR POSITION: Not prescribed.

MATERIALS OR TOOLS: Manual, rating booklet, profile form, and pencil.

METHOD: The VARS consists of 133 items representing maladaptive behavior, which are organized into six scales: Verbal Manners, Communication Skills, Attendance and Punctuality, Interpersonal Behavior, Respect for Property, Rules, and Regulations, and Grooming and Personal Hygiene. The rater records behaviors that have been observed over a specified observation period of direct contact (typically 1 month or a minimum of 70 hours). Ideally, two independent ratings of a subject should be obtained, and scoring differences averaged.

Each item is rated "Never," "Sometimes," "Often," or "Regularly" based on observed frequency of the behavior. Administration of the scales takes 30–40 minutes.

INTERPRETATION: Two scores are derived from the VARS: The frequency score reflects the occurrence of maladaptive behavior, and the severity score reflects how likely it is that the behavior would result in termination of employment. The latter is developed from employment supervisors' ratings, and while they are more subjective, they are useful in determining readiness for employment. Raw scale and total scores can be converted to percentiles and compared with the norm group. The manual also describes seven levels of employment placement and provides profiles of scores typical of each level. A positive VARS profile indicates that social behavior is sufficient for independent employment *provided job skills are adequate.*

RELIABILITY: Interrater reliability is moderate to high. Internal consistency is uniformly high as determined by correlating item scores with scale scores and total scores during sample administrations.

VALIDITY: Employment supervisors examined items for content validity. Factor analysis yielded six stable scales. Concurrent validity is exhibited by significant correlations with selected scales on the AAMD ABS and the San Francisco Vocational Competency Scale. Concurrent and predictive validity are demonstrated by placement decisions of retarded workers in sheltered workshops.

SOURCE: Published by: Western Psychological Services, 12031 Wilshire Boulevard, Los Angeles, CA 90025. Tel: 800-648-8857; Fax: 310-478-7838. (**1980**)

COST: $$

SAMPLE: <u>Interpersonal Behavior</u>	<u>Never</u>	<u>Sometimes</u>	<u>Often</u>	<u>Regularly</u>
Laughs inappropriately				
Fails to accept subordinate role				
Stops work when praised				

❑ Vocational Interest Inventory—Revised (VII-R)

AUTHOR: Patricia W. Lunneborg, PhD

FORMAT: Paper-and-pencil forced-choice questionnaire.

PURPOSE: VII-R measures students' relative interest in eight employment areas for use in vocational and educational guidance. It is most helpful for students whose interests are not yet well defined.

POPULATION: High school students. (Norms are based on 27,444 high school juniors and seniors.)

SETTING OR POSITION: Not prescribed.

MATERIALS OR TOOLS: Manual, pencil, and computer-scored test report (mail-in form or microcomputer disk).

METHOD: VII-R consists of 112 forced-choice statements of preference in Occupations (job titles) and Activities (familiar activities related to jobs). It covers Roe's eight occupational areas, which classify virtually all job types: Service, Business Contact, Organization, Technical, Outdoor, Science, General Culture, and Arts and Entertainment. Items were reviewed to eliminate sex bias and incorporate nontraditional interests. The assessment yields two scores: 8 scale scores to compare each occupational interest to the norms, and Similarity to College Majors to compare score patterns with those of college graduates. It is self-administered, individually or in groups, in 25 minutes or less and is computer scored by the publisher.

INTERPRETATION: The report provides a personalized narrative report in duplicate, with a profile of occupational interests, analysis and discussion of all scores above 75%, a profile of college student scores to compare with the subject's results, and a ranked list of college majors compatible with the subject's interests.

RELIABILITY: Internal consistency and split-half reliability are reported acceptable for the Occupations and Activities subscales (ranging .46–.72 and .37–.61 respectively) with the exception of Technical, which was less reliable. Test-retest reliability with a 3-week interval ranged from .75–.88, and with a 6-month interval ranged from .66–.85.

VALIDITY: Concurrent validity was evident in studies examining the relationship between scores and students' intended occupations, majors, and high school activities. Construct validity was demonstrated by the correspondence between college students' and vocational/technical students' majors and their high school interest scores; VII-R interest areas also correlated with Vocational Preference Inventory and Strong-Campbell Interest Inventory, corroborating the occupational classification. Predictive validity is based on the correlation of students' interest profiles with successfully completed college majors and programs.

SOURCE: Published by: Western Psychological Services, 12031 Wilshire Boulevard, Los Angeles, CA 90025. Tel: 800-648-8857; Fax: 310-478-7838. **(1993)**

COST: $$ (microcomputer disk—$$$).

SAMPLE: I would rather (A) Baby-sit (B) Talk people into voting for our schools.

I would rather learn to (A) Repair a bicycle (B) Use a microscope.

❏ Vocational Research Interest Inventory (VRII)®

AUTHORS: Vocational Research Institute (VRI) division of the Philadelphia Jewish Employment and Vocational Services (JEVS)

FORMAT: Paper and pencil, software, or scannable questionnaire.

PURPOSE: The VRII assesses interest in Department of Labor Interest Areas for early career exploration, career counseling, and transitional and community program planning. It is used in schools, work programs, correctional facilities, and other institutions to provide information on occupational interests.

POPULATION: Adolescents and adults. (Norms are based on two nationwide samples: 856 prevocational secondary school students or subjects under 18 years, and 525 vocational postsecondary students over 18 and adults in rehabilitation, job training, or other vocational counseling programs. Norms are available for the Hispanic population based on a nationwide sample representing 21 nations of origin.)

SETTING OR POSITION: Not prescribed.

MATERIALS OR TOOLS: Paper-and-pencil version: manual and test forms; software version: diskette for IBM or compatible computer; and scannable version: handbook, software for Scantron Optical Readers, item booklets, response forms, and Report Folios. An alternate paper-and-pencil form is available in Spanish.

METHOD: This self-administered 162-item questionnaire is categorized according to the 12 U.S. Department of Labor Interest Areas, written at the fourth grade reading level. The subject reads a list of vocationally oriented statements and for each item checks "LIKE", (?), or "DISLIKE." Scoring is completed by hand for the paper and pencil version, or by computer for the other two versions. (Results may be sent to VRI for scoring.) It may be administered individually or in groups and requires 15–20 minutes to administer and score. The questionnaire may be read to subjects with reading difficulty.

INTERPRETATION: Results are compared to the appropriate norm group for percentile scores. An Individual Profile Analysis statistically analyzes the relative strength of interests to determine which interest areas are highest and lowest across the 12-scale profile.

RELIABILITY: Internal consistency studies indicated high intercorrelations among the 12 interest scales (mean .86, ranging .82–.91). Test–retest reliability for 82 subjects yielded scale correlations ranging from .74–.86, with mean .83.

VALIDITY: The VRII was validated with the U.S. Employment Service Interest Inventory as the criterion demonstrating a strong relationship between the VRII and USES I.I. scores (.64–.91). Based on strong reliability and validity of the VRII, a Spanish language alternative was developed with a panel of experts from diverse Hispanic backgrounds.

SOURCE: Obtain from: Vocational Research Institute, 1528 Walnut Street, Suite 1502, Philadelphia, PA 19102. Tel: 800-VRI-JEVS. (**1985**)

COST: $—Paper-and-pencil version; $$$—software or scannable version.

SAMPLE: Not available.

❏ Vocational Transit Aptitude Battery

AUTHORS: Vocational Research Institute (VRI) division of the Philadelphia Jewish Employment and Vocational Services (JEVS)

FORMAT: Computerized multiple choice.

PURPOSE: This vocational evaluation was developed to measure perceptual and dexterity aptitudes in individuals who are mentally retarded through computer-controlled testing modules. It is designed to assess vocational capabilities for the range of jobs considered most appropriate to limited mental abilities.

POPULATION: Adolescents and adults with disabilities that involve a cognitive component, particularly moderate to severe mental retardation, but also applicable to the learning disabled or brain injured. (Three norm groups were based on 122 individuals who are developmentally disabled and 240 adults and adolescents [nonimpaired] from vocational schools and training programs.)

SETTING OR POSITION: Not prescribed.

MATERIALS OR TOOLS: Three types of dexterity test apparatus using pegs, rivets and collars, and wand; form perception book; client information checklist; manual and software. All are intended for linking to a computer, and are packaged in a portable plastic carrying case. Computer requirements are described.

METHOD: Vocational Transit has four separate components, given in order of complexity: motor coordination, manual dexterity, finger dexterity, and form perception. The three timed dexterity tests involve touching metal contacts with a wand, manually extracting, turning, and replacing pegs into holes, and completing rivet assemblies; signal lights and tones indicate correct positions or completed rows. Form perception is untimed and requires the subject to identify the stimulus form from a

multiple-choice selection; the examiner enters responses using a keypad. Each test is preceded by verbal instructions, demonstration, and practice trials with prompting as needed. The subject must reach a predetermined criterion during practice in order to take the test; thus, the learning phase is separated from performance. Assistance needed and other comments are recorded. Responses are recorded by the software program, scored by number of correct responses, and interpreted by the computer.

INTERPRETATION: Raw scores are converted to percentiles for each of three norm groups, and reported on a bar graph using a 5-point rating system for aptitudes. The computer generates a standardized report with specific test behaviors as well as scores and ratings for the four aptitudes. The aptitude scores combined with evaluator's ratings on physical demands and environmental tolerances form a profile that is compared with a database of about 800 unskilled jobs. Jobs that meet the subject's qualifications are printed out.

RELIABILITY: Test–retest reliability with a week's interval ranged from .74–.94, and from .70–.91 for a developmentally disabled sample.

VALIDITY: Vocational Transit Form Perception was validated against Apticom Form Perception (.47); dexterity scores correlated with General Aptitude Test Battery (.61–.80); and Vocational Transit aptitude scores were used as predictors of VIEWS Work Sample time scores (.87), indicating a strong relationship between work aptitude and production speed.

SOURCE: Obtain from: Vocational Research Institute, 1528 Walnut Street, Suite 1502, Philadelphia, PA 19102. Tel: 800-VRI-JEVS. **(1989)**

COST: $$$$+; training recommended.

SAMPLE: Not available.

❐ Work Adjustment Inventory: Measures of Job-Related Temperament (WAI)

AUTHOR: James E. Gilliam

FORMAT: Norm-referenced self-report

PURPOSE: This assessment of work-related temperament helps to determine whether a worker has the temperament needed for a job and for getting along with other workers. It is designed for use in schools, clinics, and research, and can assist in recommending job placement as well as individual transitional plans for students with disabilities.

POPULATION: Adolescents and adults, ages 12–22 years, who are just beginning to work. (Standardization sample consisted of 7,399 students, 10% with disabilities, representative of the 1990 U.S. population.)

SETTING OR POSITION: Comfortable room with minimal distractions, adequate lighting and ventilation, and a place to sit and take the test.

MATERIALS OR TOOLS: Manual, Response Record Form, and a pencil.

METHOD: WAI is an 80-item self-report consisting of short positive statements about how the subject perceives himself or herself. Each item is rated on a 5-point scale from almost never to almost always. The items are categorized in six scales measuring six work-related temperament traits: Activity, Empathy, Sociability, Assertiveness, Adaptability, and Emotionality. The scores on the six scales are totalled, then added together to obtain an overall score. The WAI may be administered individually or in groups, requiring approximately 15–20 minutes. The examiner may record responses for a subject who is unable to do so.

INTERPRETATION: Each scale yields a percentile rank and standard score for age and gender, offering a Profile of Standard Scores that indicates how well the subject will fit in with other workers and with the task requirements. (Descriptive paragraphs in the manual elaborate on the interpretation of scores in each scale.) Standard scores are totalled together for an overall quotient score of work temperament and adjustment.

RELIABILITY: Internal consistency coefficients are reported adequate (82% of total test scores $\geq$ .90, and 21% of scale scores $\geq$ .90, 49% $\geq$ .80, and 90% $\geq$ .70). Test–retest reliability with a 2-week interval was .80 for WAI quotient, ranging from .72–.89 for the scale scores, all significant at .01 level.

VALIDITY: Content validity is based on review of literature on temperament, review of existing temperament tests, clinical experience, and consultation with experts in vocational rehabilitation. Factor analysis of the data produced the six factors on which the scales are based. Student WAI scores correlated modestly (.39) with scores by outside raters on the Job Performance Questionnaire. The construct that temperament traits are stable over time is supported by their constancy across all ages. Construct validity is further supported by the significant correlations (.32–.83) of all scales with the WAI quotient.

SOURCE: Available from: Pro-Ed, 8700 Shoal Creek Boulevard, Austin, TX 78757-0603. Tel: 800-FXPROED; Fax: 512-451-8542. (**1994**)

COST: $$

SAMPLE: I like to start off on my own and keep going.   1 2 3 4 5

I don't mind being told what to do.   1 2 3 4 5

❐ Worker Role Interview (WRI) (Research Version)

AUTHORS: Craig Velozo, PhD, OTR/L, Gary Kielhofner, DrPH, OTR, FAOTA, and Gail Fisher, MPA, OTR/L

FORMAT: Semi-structured interview and rating scale.

PURPOSE: The interview is intended as the psychosocial/environmental component of the injured worker's initial rehabilitation assessment. Combined with observations made during other physical and behavioral assessment procedures, it is designed to identify specific variables influencing the subject's ability to return to work. The WRI is part of a larger database research project studying the ability of low back pain clients to return to work.

POPULATION: Work-hardening clients with physical disabilities (low back pain, hand injuries); an unpublished study developed a version for psychiatric clients (Kielhofner, 1995).

SETTING OR POSITION: Any relevant setting is permitted.

MATERIALS OR TOOLS: Manual and rating forms, pencil.

METHOD: The interview covers various aspects of the subject's life and job setting associated with past work experience. The authors describe WRI in the context of five comprehensive steps: (1) prepare for the interview (determine client is appropriate and gather preliminary data); (2) conduct interview at the beginning of the initial assessment (28 recommended questions provided); (3) complete physical/work capacity assessment procedures usually conducted at the facility; (4) score initial evaluation with comments using 4-point rating scale based on the Model of Human Occupation; and (5) record discharge evaluation scores and comments based on impressions of completed rehabilitation (interview is not repeated). The rating form contains six content areas divided into subcontent areas that influence return to work. It yields 17 ratings based on specific scoring criteria. Administration requires 30–60 minutes and 10–15 minutes for scoring.

INTERPRETATION: The Initial and Discharge ratings are plotted on a single rating form to obtain a profile of the subject. Ratings range from 4 (findings strongly support client returning to employment) to 1 (findings significantly interfere with client returning to employment). The administrator must determine whether to score the WRI for return to previous employment or to employment in general. Comments comprise the issues or reasons on which the ratings are based.

RELIABILITY: Test–retest reliability with a 6- to 12-day interval was .95 for total score, with a range of .86–.94 for the six content areas. Interrater reliability for 3 raters scoring each of 30 adult rehabilitation subjects with upper extremity injuries was .81 (ranging .46–.92 for six content areas), indicating further refinement is necessary (Biernacki, 1993). Further studies are in progress.

VALIDITY: The subcontent areas are derived from an extensive literature review of factors that seem to influence return to work. An unpublished study supports construct validity. Further studies are in progress.

SOURCES: Distributed by: Model of Human Occupation Clearinghouse, University of Illinois at Chicago, Department of Occupational Therapy (M/C 811), College of Associated Health Professions, 1919 West Taylor Street, Chicago, IL 60612-7250. Tel: 312-996-6901; Fax: 312-413-0256. (**1992**)

Biernacki, S. (1993). Reliability of the Worker Role Interview. *American Journal of Occupational Therapy, 47*, 797–803.

Kielhofner, G. (1995). *A model of human occupation:*

Theory and application (2nd edition). Baltimore: Williams & Wilkins.

COST: $

SAMPLE: How has your injury affected you outside of work? (H = habits)

How did you choose your present job? (V = volition)

Do you think you were good at your job before your injury? (PC = personal causation)

Play

Assessments

❏ Children's Playfulness Scale (CPS)

AUTHOR: Lynn A. Barnett, revised from original by J. Lieberman

FORMAT: Rating scale based on observations and impressions.

PURPOSE: The scale identifies and measures the quality of playfulness, or the internal predisposition to be playful, as manifested in everyday play behavior. This method of assessing play is purported by Barnett to be more productive than focusing on specific play behaviors and interactions.

POPULATION: Preschool and toddler-aged children. (Sample consisted of 388 children, ages 29–61.5 months, from 7 daycare centers.)

SETTING OR POSITION: Not prescribed.

MATERIALS OR TOOLS: Questionnaire and pencil.

METHOD: The instrument consists of 23 item statements categorized into 5 component playfulness dimensions: physical spontaneity, social spontaneity, cognitive spontaneity, manifest joy, and sense of humor. Raters use observation and knowledge of the children to rate them along a 5-point scale, from "sounds exactly like the child" to "doesn't sound at all like the child." Barnett recommends that the examiner have some background and experience with young children as well as a minimum of 30 hours of observing the child's playful style across situations and contexts.

INTERPRETATION: The CPS yields a total playfulness score as well as a profile of dimension scores, providing a conceptual and methodological way of viewing play. Rather than measuring specific behaviors or physical characteristics of the setting, it examines the child's underlying predisposition to bring a playful quality to interactions with the environment (including people, places, and things).

RELIABILITY: Interrater reliability coefficients were .92 (test session), .96 (1-month retest), and .97 (3-month retest). Ratings by students were also reliable (.94). Test–retest reliabilities were ..84–.88 for 1-month interval, .88–.92 for 3-month interval, and .89–.95 between the two retests. Internal consistency reliabilities ranged from .80–.89 for the 5 dimensions, .88 for the total scale, .63–.71 for correlations between playfulness factors, and .72–.79 between factors and total playfulness score.

VALIDITY: Content validity is based on literature review and review of items by panels of experts. Factor analysis confirmed 6 underlying playfulness factors: the 5 dimensions and a general playfulness factor. High convergent and low discriminant coefficients demonstrated that a frequency rating format ("almost always" to "almost never") has similar factorial validity to the extent rating format used. Construct validity was demonstrated by correlations generalized to non–daycare samples, ages 26.75 to 62.25 months, and by comparison of CPS to other play measures (Lieberman's original playfulness scale, Child Behaviors Inventory of Playfulness, and Rubin's Play Observation Scale).

SOURCES: Found in: Barnett, L.A. Playfulness: Definition, design, and measurement. *Play & Culture*, 3, 319–336. (**1990**)

Barnett, L.A. (1991). The playful child: Measurement of a disposition to play. *Play & Culture*, 4, 51–74.

Leiberman, J. (1977). *Playfulness: Its relationship to imagination and creativity.* New York: Academic Press.

COST: ¢

SAMPLE: Sense of humor
> The child enjoys joking with other children.
> The child gently teases others while at play.

❐ Play History

AUTHOR: Nancy Takata, MA, OTR

FORMAT: Semistructured interview.

PURPOSE: This tool is designed to identify a child's play experiences and play opportunities. In measuring the qualitative and quantitative dimensions of play, it can be used for diagnostic as well as treatment planning purposes.

POPULATION: Children and adolescents. (Sample for the original 1969 version was 23 outpatients, ages 1.7 to 19.5 years, representing a cross-section of multihandicapping conditions and socioeconomic backgrounds and cultures.)

SETTING OR POSITION: Home or clinical setting.

MATERIALS OR TOOLS: Not prescribed; presumed to be common contents of the play environment.

METHOD: The Play History (Takata, 1974) has three sections: general information, previous play experiences (arranged in developmental sequence), and actual play examination (including a recent 3-day sampling or play schedule). The latter two categories each consist of nine subcategories for describing the form and content of the play behavior. Data are gained from a primary caregiver of the child and are analyzed and charted according to a play taxonomy (describing five epochs in play development from sensorimotor to recreation). Four elements are highlighted: materials, action, people, and setting. The history yields a description of the play. The description in Takata's original article in 1969 differs in form and content: It consists of a two-part questionnaire, yielding descriptive data on the qualitative and quantitative nature of play, according to seven play factors.

INTERPRETATION: The instrument yields a total play description of the child for detecting children with play dysfunctions and for planning and evaluating treatment. Assets and deficits of the child's play are identified, resulting in a play prescription.

RELIABILITY: Interrater reliability of videotaped interviews was .91 (nonhandicapped sample higher than handicapped sample), with category scores significant at .58–.85. Test–retest reliability with a 3-week interval was .77 for overall score and ranging .41–.78 for categories, with suggestions to improve reliability of caregiver responses. (The author cautions the examiner to develop skill in history taking.)

VALIDITY: Content validity is based on extensive literature review. Concurrent validity is demonstrated by: correlation with Minnesota Child Development Inventory (overall score .97 for nondisabled, .70 for disabled, most category correlations above .70); correlation of epoch scores with age (.85, with .94 for nondisabled and .79 for disabled); and significant difference in scores between disabled and nondisabled, suggesting impeded development among the disabled.

SOURCES: Found in: Behnke, C., & Fetkovich, M. Examining the reliability and validity of the Play History, *American Journal of Occupational Therapy, 38,* 94–100. (**1984**)

Takata, N. (1974). Play as a prescription. In M. Reilly (Ed.), *Play as exploratory learning*(pp.209–246). Beverly Hills, CA: Sage Publications.

Takata, N. (1969). The play history. *American Journal of Occupational Therapy, 23,* 314–318.

COST: ¢

SAMPLE: Actual Play Examination
<u>How</u> does the child play with toys and other materials?
<u>What body postures</u> does the child use during play?

❐ Play Observation

AUTHOR: Alex F. Kalverboer

FORMAT: Rating system using videotaped behavior in standardized setting.

PURPOSE: This instrument is a method of gathering data on children's behavior (play and other) in standardized conditions. It provides a detailed description of behavior relative to the social and physical environment, as well as to the child's own body.

POPULATION: Appropriate for children with neurobehavioral problems in language, social communication, motor ability, or attention. (Sample consisted of 147 preschool children, ages 4.10–5.4 years, randomly selected from full-term babies born in a single hospital.)

SETTING OR POSITION: Specially designed playroom, with block pattern on the floor, structured differently for each of the six recordings.

MATERIALS, OR TOOLS: Videorecorder, protocol sheets for scoring, and specified variety of blocks and toys.

METHOD: Videotaped recordings are made of six standardized sessions, ranging from 3 to 15 minutes each and totalling 39 minutes. In each, the child is either alone or with mother or observer and with or without toys. The tapes are then viewed and carefully scored by two observers, according to engagement in any of 12 behaviors, 5 levels of complexity in play, and other characteristics of play and activity level. The record is detailed down to 10-second segments.

INTERPRETATION: The instrument yields a profile of scores in the 12 areas rated, as well as duration, frequency, and levels of play.

Reliability: Interrater reliability ranges from .73 to .91 for each item; test–retest on ratings 6 weeks apart is .73 to .99.

VALIDITY: Concurrent validity is based on low correlations with intelligence scores (.14 to .27).

SOURCE: Kalverboer, A. A measurement of play: Clinical applications. In B. Tizard & D. Harvey (Eds.), *Biology of play.* Philadelphia: Lippincott. (1977)

COST: ¢

SAMPLE: Play Activity Level I: Play activities that are not specific to the material handled and that have no observable constructive or symbolic character.

❑ Preschool Play Scale, Revised

AUTHOR: Susan H. Knox, MA, OTR, FAOTA

FORMAT: Observation-based rating tool.

PURPOSE: This observational assessment is designed to provide a developmental description of typical play behavior. The instrument is useful in identifying interest areas, determining treatment effectiveness, and evaluating children who cannot cooperate with standardized tests.

POPULATION: Children 0–6 years. (Pilot sample consisted of 12 preschool children with mental retardation. Further studies demonstrate use with a variety of nondisabled and disabled population samples.)

SETTING OR POSITION: Naturalistic or familiar environments, both indoors and outdoors, with peers present.

MATERIALS OR TOOLS: Not prescribed; a variety of play materials should be available.

METHOD: The instrument was originally organized by yearly increments in four dimensions: space management, material management, imitation, and participation. Knox's proposed revision incorporates 6-month increments to age 3, replaces the imitation dimension with pretense/symbolic (which includes imitation), and revises item descriptions, scoring, and administration. The dimensions are made up of 12 factors, which are defined by behavior descriptors. The child is observed during free play for a minimum of two 30-minute periods, indoors and outdoors. The descriptors are marked every time they are observed. Each factor is then ranked at the highest incremental level at which the child behaves. Dimension scores are the mean of their factor scores; the overall play age is the mean of the dimension scores.

INTERPRETATION: The score describes play maturity (= play age) and is determined by the highest level of behavior demonstrated for each dimension. The overall play age is a stable estimate of the child's play maturity, and correlates with the child's developmental age. In addition, item scores can indicate specific strengths and weaknesses.

RELIABILITY: All research is based on the original version. Bledsoe and Shephard examined reliability on normal preschoolers, finding interrater reliability to range from .89 to .93 for category scores, .98 for the dimensions, and .996 for overall play age (the authors were the two raters); test–retest reliability ranged from .67 to .91 for category scores and .85 to .97 for dimensions and play age scores. Harrison and Kielhofner, testing handicapped children, reported satisfactory interrater (.88) and test–retest (.91) reliability.

VALIDITY: Content validity is based on play theory literature. Scores were found to discriminate among chronological ages (.996 and .74 correlations). Concurrent validity is demonstrated by correlation of scores with play scales by Lunzer (.64, .59) and Parten (.61, .60) in the two studies by Bledsoe and Shephard (1982) and Harrison and Kielhofner (1986). Additional studies demonstrated score differences among groups with various handicapping conditions, and following intervention.

SOURCES: Found in: Knox, S. Development and current use of the Knox Preschool Play Scale. In D. Parham & L. Fazio (Eds.), *Play: A clinical focus in occupational therapy for children*. St. Louis, MO: Mosby Yearbooks. (**in press**)

Bledsoe, N.P., & Shephard, J.T. (1982). A study of reliability and validity of a preschool play scale. *American Journal of Occupational Therapy, 36*, 783–788.

Harrison, H., & Kielhofner, G. (1986). Examining reliability of Preschool Play Scale with handicapped children. *American Journal of Occupational Therapy, 40,* 167–173.

COST: ¢

SAMPLE: Material Management (18–24 months)

Manipulation: operates mechanical toy, pulls apart pop beads, strings beads

Construction: uses tools

Purpose: foresight before acting

Attention: quiet play 5–10 minutes; play with single object 5 min.

❑ Test of Playfulness (ToP)

AUTHOR: Anita Bundy, ScD, OTR, FAOTA

FORMAT: Observation-based behavior rating scale.

PURPOSE: By observing children engaged in free play, the occupation of play is assessed by the individual's *playfulness* rather than by the cognitive, motor, or language skills the child uses in play or by the activity in which the child engages.

POPULATION: Designed for typically developing children ages 15 months through 10 years, regardless of disability. (Pilot sample is based on 200 children throughout the U.S. and Toronto.)

SETTING OR POSITION: Familiar play settings, indoors and outdoors, with familiar playmates present.

MATERIALS OR TOOLS: Familiar toys or objects that can be used in play (natural or fabricated) should be available. For very young children (less than 2 years), a familiar caregiver should play with the child, following the child's lead.

METHOD: The ToP consists of 68 items, each reflecting a defined behavioral trait. The traits represent four elements of playfulness: intrinsic motivation, internal control, disengagement from constraints of reality, and framing. The child is observed by a trained examiner during a 15-minute play period (both indoors and outdoors) and rated on as many as 3 playfulness scales: extent, intensity, and skillfulness. The ratings range from 0 (lowest) to 3 (highest).

INTERPRETATION: Standard scores are not yet available. Development of the assessment through Rasch analysis is in progress, however the raw scores can be used cautiously to create a playfulness profile. Each of the four elements is portrayed by a continuum. Scores are plotted on the continuum, describing the child's position on each continuum. The cumulative contribution of each element determines the child's relative playfulness (also on a continuum).

RELIABILITY: Preliminary evidence of interrater reliability is exhibited by the 1995 pilot study in which 100% of trained raters fit the Rasch model (i.e., assigned ratings in expected ways, demonstrating consistency relative to other raters).

VALIDITY: Preliminary construct validity is demonstrated by the 1995 pilot study, in which 96% of children and 94% of items fit the Rasch model. Additional pilot studies and a concurrent validity study are in progress.

SOURCES: Available from the author at: Department of Occupational Therapy , Colorado State University, Room 219, Occupational Therapy Building, Fort Collins, CO: 80523. Tel: 970-491-6253. (**revised 1993**)

Partial description found in : Parham, L.D. (Ed.). (in press). *Play in occupational therapy*. St. Louis, MO: Mosby Yearbooks.

COST: ¢; raters must be trained and contribute data toward test development.

SAMPLE:	ITEM	EXT	INT	SKILL	COMMENTS
	Appears to feel safe.				
	Initiates play with others.				

❏ Transdisciplinary Play-Based Assessment (TPBA)

AUTHOR: Toni W. Linder, EdD

FORMAT: Questionnaire and rating form based on observation of unstructured and structured performance (nonstandardized).

PURPOSE: This nonstandardized holistic instrument uses natural play interactions for a comprehensive assessment of the child's development and underlying developmental processes, learning style, interaction patterns, and other behaviors. It identifies strengths and needs, determines eligibility of the child for services, and recommends intervention and curriculum strategies.

POPULATION: Children functioning between infancy and 6 years, with or without disabilities.

SETTING OR POSITION: A well-equipped large room arranged with distinct play areas visible to the child, with a one-way mirror or corner of the room set aside for observers. A preschool classroom is optimal, but any creative play environment may be used, including the child's home.

MATERIALS OR TOOLS: The room should be arranged with toys and materials to encourage play and to facilitate exploratory, manipulative, and problem-solving behaviors, emotional expression, and language skills. Recommendations are given.

METHOD: The assessment is organized into five domains of development: cognitive, social–emotional, communication and language, and sensorimotor. TPBA uses a team approach of collaborative observation, which includes the child's parents. Its nontechnical language is understandable to both lay and professional persons. Parents first complete developmental checklists about the child's performance level at home, which is used to plan a play session. An interdisciplinary team then observes the child for 1 1/2 hours during play

activities with a play facilitator, parents, and a peer; the facilitator encourages optimal performance with enticing toys and play strategies. (Videotaping the session is desirable.) The session comprises six phases: unstructured facilitation (child leads, facilitator follows and expands), structured facilitation, introduction of peer to observe interaction, unstructured and structured play with parents (including separation from parents), unstructured and structured motor play, and snack (for oral–motor and other observations). The format allows for flexibility in content, participants, and sequence based on the needs of the child. Observation worksheets are completed according to TPBA guidelines, following discussion and analysis of the child's developmental level, learning style, interaction patterns, and other behaviors. The summary sheet describes the child's strengths, rating of abilities, justification of the ratings, and interdisciplinary recommendations.

INTERPRETATION: The assessment yields a comprehensive and detailed individualized report and program plan for the child and family, including developmental level of the child, family assessment, intervention services, and optimum environment. A companion text, *Transdisciplinary Play-Based Intervention: Guidelines for Developing a Meaningful Curriculum for Young Children*, offers a play-based approach to intervention based on TPBA results, including team ideas for play linking program objectives to home intervention and classroom curriculum. TPBA can serve for ongoing review and evaluation of the intervention.

RELIABILITY: Studies are in progress, according to the author.

VALIDITY: Content validity is apparent from the review of literature and existing tests, and from consultation with teachers, therapists, and parents. Further studies are in progress.

SOURCE: Linder, T.W. *Transcisciplinary play-based assessment: A functional approach to working with young children, revised edition*, Baltimore: Paul H. Brookes. (**1993**)

COST: $

SAMPLE: Social–Emotional Observation Worksheet

Social Interactions with Peers

A. In dyad

   1. Acknowledgment of peer *(circle those that apply)*:

     a. Ignoring, withdrawing, unaware

     b. Looking at, watching

     c. Touching, gesturing

     d. Vocalizing toward, talking with peer

   Examples:

Leisure

Assessments

❏ Activity Index: Activity Patterns and Leisure Concepts Among the Elderly (Nystrom)/Occupational Behavior and Life Satisfaction Among Retirees (Gregory)

AUTHORS: E. P. Nystrom and Mark D. Gregory

FORMAT: Structured interview (Nystrom); self-report questionnaire (Gregory).

PURPOSE: Both instruments examine the meaning and significance of activity and activity patterns among the elderly. Gregory adapted Nystrom's tool for use with retirees.

POPULATION: Elderly, age 65 and over. (Nystrom's study took place in a low income housing development; Gregory's subjects resided in rest homes or retirement communities or belonged to senior centers or a social or church group.)

SETTING OR POSITION: Not prescribed.

MATERIALS OR TOOLS: Interview format (Nystrom); questionnaire and pencil (Gregory).

METHOD: Nystrom's interview contains 61 questions on activity, leisure, and the meaning of leisure, including rating the degree of participation in 25 stated activities and ideal leisure preferences. In Gregory's questionnaire, activities are rated according to degree of enjoyment, internal versus external motivation, and sense of competence.

INTERPRETATION: Both instruments yield a summed score for participation in activities, as well as listings of preferred activities. With respect to meaning of activities, Nystrom's tool yields descriptive data while Gregory's yields a summed score.

RELIABILITY: Nystrom demonstrates interrater (.73) and internal reliability. Gregory demonstrates test–retest at .70 for Part 1, .87 for Part 2, and .72 for Part 3 with split-half reliability at .90.

VALIDITY: Nystrom: content and concurrent validity reported. Gregory: concurrent with other measures of life satisfaction, adjustment, and morale.

SOURCES: Gregory, M.D. Occupational behavior and life satisfaction among retirees. *American Journal of Occupational Therapy, 37,* 548–553. (**1983**)

Nystrom, E.P. (1974). Activity patterns and leisure concepts among the elderly. *American Journal of Occupational Therapy, 28,* 337–345.

COST: ¢

SAMPLE: For every activity check: don't do, not interested/would like to; do at least once a week/3 times a week.

❑ Interest Checklist

AUTHORS: Janice Matsutsuyu; revised by Joan Rogers, PhD, OTR, Jennifer Weinstein, OTR, LPT, and Joanne Firone, MA, OTR (additional modifications on this version available from source below)

FORMAT: Questionnaire (self-administered) and interview.

PURPOSE: The checklist gathers data about a person's interest patterns and characteristics, which give a perspective of interest involvement over a lifetime.

POPULATION: The tool was developed for adults but has been found useful for adolescence through old age. (It was originally tested on psychiatric inpatients at the Neuropsychiatric Institute [NPI] at UCLA.)

SETTING OR POSITION: Not prescribed.

MATERIALS OR TOOLS: Checklist and pencil.

METHOD: The instrument consists of three parts: an 80-item checklist (with degree of interest indicated), a section to indicate additional interests, and a section requesting a narrative of leisure interest history (written or by interview). The checklist portion was modified by Rogers, Weinstein, and Firone (1978), changing the degree of interest to a 5-point rating scale and disputing the classification of the interest categories according to their factor analysis. The tool yields a list of interests that can be logically categorized into either classification system. Depending on the breadth of the interview, descriptive information can be obtained about the subject's past experiences, present resources and constraints, and the role of interests in guiding the subject's behavior. A modified checklist of 68 items recommended for use with the Model of Human Occupation (MOHO) is available from the MOHO Clearinghouse (see source).

INTERPRETATION: The interests identified by the subject can be used in treatment planning and can be compared to subject's capabilities, roles, and patterns of activity in determining the need for modification.

RELIABILITY: Test–retest reliability with 3-week interval is good (.92, with range of .84–.92 for each category) for the version by Rogers et al.

VALIDITY: Face validity is evident. Rogers et al. disagreed with the classification of interests and reclassified them according to their own factor analysis. Hemphill (1988) summarized studies in which the Checklist discriminates among normal and diagnostic groups (alcoholic, medical, psychiatric, mentally retarded).

SOURCES: Modified Interest Checklist available from: Model of Human Occupation Clearinghouse, Department of Occupational Therapy (M/C 811), College of Associated Health Professions, 1919 W. Taylor Street, Chicago, IL 60612-7250. Tel: 312-996-6901; Fax: 312-413-0256.

Matsutsuyu, J. The Interest Checklist. *American Journal of Occupational Therapy, 11,* 179–181. (**1967**)

Rogers, J., Weinstein, J., & Firone, J. (1978). The Interest Checklist: An empirical assessment. *American Journal of Occupational Therapy, 32,* 628–630.

Rogers, J.C. (1988). The NPI interest checklist. In B. Hemphill (Ed.), *Mental health assessments in occupational therapy* (pp. 93–114). Thorofare, NJ: Slack.

COST: ¢

SAMPLE:	Activity	Interest
	Gardening	Casual—strong—no

❏ Leisure Activities Blank

AUTHOR: George E. McKechnie

FORMAT: Paired rating scales, self-report.

PURPOSE: This tool is designed to gather information on past leisure activities and to predict future satisfaction with these activities. The author suggests it is useful for individuals forced to change leisure pursuits (as in illness).

POPULATION: Adults and elderly. (Initial sample consisted of 288 affluent adults over 20 years, living in a geography and climate favorable for recreation.)

SETTING OR POSITION: Not prescribed.

MATERIALS OR TOOLS: The two scales.

METHOD: The instrument consists of a list of 121 activities currently popular in the U.S. They fall into seven categories: mechanics, crafts, intellectual, slow living, neighborhood sports, glamour sports, and fast living. On the first scale, the subject rates his or her past participation in each activity (from 1 to 4), and future intentions to participate (from 1 to 3) on the second scale. (Morgan and Godbey [1978] altered the second scale to present participation, to indicate current activity changes.)

INTERPRETATION: The tool yields 14 scores: seven for past participation in each category and seven for future intentions in each category.

RELIABILITY: Split-half reliability is good for each subscale. Test–retest reliability with 3-week interval is good (mean .83 for past scales and .85 for future scales).

VALIDITY: Factor analysis clearly identified the seven categories. Concurrent with environmental dispositions; sensitive to changes in environmental circumstances.

SOURCES: Published by: Consulting Psychologists Press, 577 College Ave., Palo Alto, CA 94306. Tel: 800-624-1765; Fax: 415-969-8608. (**1975**)

Morgan, A., & Godbey, G. (1978). The effect of entering an age-segregated environment upon the leisure activity pattern of older adults. *Journal of Leisure Research, 10,* 77–190.

COST: $

SAMPLE: Permission to reprint sample item not granted.

❏ Self-Assessment of Leisure Interests

AUTHOR: Lisette N. Kautzmann, EdD, OTR, FAOTA

FORMAT: Checklist.

PURPOSE: This interest checklist is designed to identify and encourage interest in leisure activities that are safe and within the capabilities of arthritic individuals. The self-assessment format is based on Knowles' self-diagnostic competency model to maximize subject's responsibility in evaluation and treatment planning.

POPULATION: Adults with arthritis.

SETTING OR POSITION: Not prescribed.

MATERIALS OR TOOLS: Checklist and pencil.

METHOD: The checklist consists of 71 activities divided into 8 categories (e.g., games, sports, educational, and organizational activities). Respondents rate the importance of the activity to them, level of skill or interest, and priority for future development and participation.

INTERPRETATION: The test yields a grid of checks indicating interest and involvement. The author reports that clients feel empowered by the results to pursue activities of their choice (per telephone communication with author).

RELIABILITY: No research due to the self-report format; author reports reliability may be affected by subject's mood, energy level, and pain at any given time.

VALIDITY: Face and content validity are based on literature review (screening the activity list to remove items contraindicated for individuals with arthritis) and review by a panel of experts in occupational therapy treatment of rheumatic disease.

SOURCES: Obtain from: Lisette Kautzmann, Eastern Kentucky University, Dizney 103, Richmond, KY 40475. Tel: 606-622-3300.

Kautzmann, L. (1984). Identifying leisure interests: A self-assessment approach for adults with arthritis. *Occupational Therapy in Health Care, 1*(2), 45–52.

COST: ¢

SAMPLE: Nature Activities: Gardening
Caring for house plants
Flower arranging

PERFORMANCE COMPONENTS

Sensory Awareness and

Sensory Integration

Assessments

❏ DeGangi–Berk Test of Sensory Integration

AUTHORS: Ronald A. Berk, PhD, and Georgia A. DeGangi, MS, OTR

FORMAT: Performance rating scale.

PURPOSE: The test is designed to measure sensory integration in preschoolers and to detect early sensory integrative dysfunction. It may be used for diagnostic or screening purposes.

POPULATION: Preschool children, ages 3 to 5 years. (Sample consisted of 101 normal and 30 delayed children from the Washington, DC metropolitan area and 8 delayed children from a child development center in Indiana.)

SETTING OR POSITION: Space at least 10 x 15 feet in size.

MATERIALS OR TOOLS: Child-size table and chair, tape, pencil, stopwatch, specified wood dowel and rolling pin, scooter board, hula hoop, mat, and test kit.

METHOD: The test consists of 36 items, divided into three subtests: postural control, bilateral motor integration, and reflex integration. It is administered individually in approximately 30 minute segments. Standard instructions must be followed in sequence and each item scored according to well-defined criteria. The overall score is totalled from the three subscores.

INTERPRETATION: The test yields a profile of the child's functioning level, indicating whether the performance is in the normal range or deficient.

RELIABILITY: Interrater reliability for total scores is .73 and .79 for two pairs of raters. Test–retest reliability ranged from .85 to .96 over 1-week intervals. Reliability of the Reflex Integration subtest alone is weak.

VALIDITY: Content validity is based on ratings by a panel of experts. Construct validity is based on scores discriminating between normal and delayed subjects, as well as correlation of item to test scores.

SOURCE: Published by: Western Psychological Services, 12031 Wilshire Boulevard, Los Angeles, CA 90025. Tel: 800-648-8857; Fax: 310-478-7838. (**1983**)

COST: $$

SAMPLE: "Let's do a wheelbarrow walk. I'll pick up your feet and you walk with your hands. See how far you can go."

❑ Infant/Toddler Symptom Checklist; A Screening Tool for Parents

AUTHORS: Georgia A. DeGangi, PhD, OTL, FAOTA, Susan Poisson, MA, Ruth Z. Sickel, PhD, and Andrea Santman Wiener, MHS, PT, PCS

FORMAT: Criterion-referenced screening checklist.

PURPOSE: This instrument was developed for use by parents or professionals for early identification of sensory and regulatory disorders. It can be used diagnostically to examine predispositions toward developing sensory integrative disorders; attention deficits; and emotional, behavioral, or learning difficulties. It was designed as a clinical and research tool.

POPULATION: Infants and toddlers from 7-30 months. (Two samples consisted of 154 normal and 67 infants with regulatory disorders, i.e., infants with difficulties related to sleep, self-consoling, feeding, or hyperarousal.)

SETTING OR POSITION: Not prescribed.

MATERIALS OR TOOLS: Carrying portfolio, which includes manual and scoresheets; and a pencil.

METHOD: The checklist contains 6 versions: a short 21-item general screen and 5 screens that are age specific by months. They are derived from 57 items that measure responses in the following domains: self-regulation, attention, modulation of sleep–wake states, responses to sensory stimulation, attachment, and emotional functioning. The age-specific screens should be used when possible. Accompanying the checklist is a cover sheet describing the purpose of the test and rating the infant's behaviors (never or sometimes = 0 points, most times = 2 points, past = 1 point) by the parent or by interview with the parent. Points are added up to obtain the total score on the Protocol sheet which contains scoring guidelines and interpretation (normal and deficient ranges). The checklist should be administered in one sitting in about 10 minutes. The authors recommend additional companion tests when used for diagnostic purposes.

INTERPRETATION: A total checklist score at or above the cutoff score for the age group is considered at risk for a regulatory disorder, and further diagnosis is indicated.

RELIABILITY: No information.

VALIDITY: Construct validity is demonstrated by the selection of items that discriminate between the normal subjects and subjects with regulatory disorders. Total scores accurately differentiated between the two groups, with low rates of false-delay or false-normal errors. Concurrent validity studies showed low correlations between Symptom Checklist scores and other infant tests, indicating the distinct nature of the checklist.

SOURCE: Published by: Therapy Skill Builders, a division of Psychological Corporation, 555 Academic Court, San Antonio, TX 78204-2498. Tel: 800-228-0752; Fax: 800-232-1223. (**1995**)

COST: $

SAMPLE: 1. Self-Regulation

> A. Is frequently irritable, fussy
> B. Goes easily from whimper to intense cry
> C. Can't calm self effectively by sucking on pacifier, looking at toys, or listening to caregiver

❐ McGill Pain Questionnaire (MPQ)

AUTHOR: Ronald Melzack, PhD

FORMAT: Paper-and-pencil questionnaire and structured interview.

PURPOSE: The questionnaire provides a consistent method of measuring subjective pain experience. It is designed to help subjects describe their pain, and to study the effects of pain management techniques on the quality and intensity of pain.

POPULATION: Patients with pain, assumed to be adults by the vocabulary of the questionnaire. (Sample consisted of 297 patients with numerous medical and surgical diagnoses.)

SETTING OR POSITION: Not specified.

MATERIALS OR TOOLS: Questionnaire and pencil.

METHOD: The Questionnaire consists of three groups of pain descriptor words (sensory, affective, and evaluative, plus miscellaneous words), and front and back body drawings to describe location of pain. The pain descriptors are divided into sets of words describing types of pain, with the words ranked according to degree of pain within the set. Subjects are instructed to check every word that describes their pain, and to indicate the location of the pain by shading the body figures. Each word is given a numerical value for scoring according to its rank in the set. The questionnaire requires 5–20 minutes. Melzack (1975) offers an admission version, pre- and post-procedure version, and a home recording card.

INTERPRETATION: The MPQ yields three types of measures: the pain rating index (PRI) based on the sum of the rank values of all the word sets, the total number of words chosen (NWC), and the present pain intensity (PPI), which is an overall intensity rating on a scale of 0 (no pain) to 5 (excruciating). The resulting data represent a quantitative index of pain and indicate the extent of change in the quality and intensity of pain, particularly when administered before and after a procedure or treatment modality.

RELIABILITY: Test–retest studies were summarized in which repeated administrations of the questionnaire to patients yielded consistencies of 75% and 70.3% (mean); and pain recall was assessed after intervals of 1 or 5 days, indicating highly consistent score profiles on retrospective pain reports. Intercorrelations among descriptor categories and among the three indices are highly significant.

VALIDITY: Studies of item and factor analysis yielded the list of descriptor words and the categorization into subclasses, rank values, and dimensions. Construct validity studies confirm Melzack's postulated sensory and affective dimensions, with the evaluative dimension less consistent. Affective scores correspond with scores on depression scales and predict results on Minnesota Multiphasic Personality Inventory profiles. Numerous concurrent validity studies report associations between MPQ scores and analgesia requirements, recovery from oral surgery, and other methods of pain reporting. Finally, MPQ results discriminate among specific acute versus chronic pain groups as well as other clinical pain syndromes.

SOURCES: Melzack, R. The McGill Pain Questionnaire: Major properties and scoring methods. *Pain*, 1, 277–299. (1975)

Melzack, R. (1983). *Pain measurement and assessment.* New York: Raven Press.

COST: ¢

SAMPLE: 1   FLICKERING
QUIVERING
PULSING
THROBBING
BEATING
POUNDING

❑ Pain Apperception Test (PAT)

AUTHOR: Donald V. Petrovich, PhD

FORMAT: Paper-and-pencil projective test and rating scale.

PURPOSE: In order to better understand the individual's reaction to pain, PAT was developed to evaluate the psychological variables involved in the experience of pain. It may be used for investigation into the various aspects of pain and their relationships, attitudes, and reactions to treatment procedures, and differences in pain perception among groups.

POPULATION: Adults (norms are provided for four groups: 50 male hospital personnel, 50 female hospital personnel, 100 male hospitalized veterans, and 100 males with chronic schizophrenia).

SETTING OR POSITION: Not prescribed.

MATERIALS OR TOOLS: Kit contains a manual, set of picture cards, and protocol sheets; and a pencil.

METHOD: Based on the premise that individuals perceive pain in others based on their own experiences and reactions (that is, apperception), PAT uses pictures of persons in pain to elicit a judgment of intensity and duration of the pain depicted. The test consists of 25 Picture Cards categorized in three series, each reflecting a type of pain situation: felt pain sensation, anticipation versus felt-sensation of pain (i.e., imminent infliction versus already inflicted), and self-inflicted versus other-inflicted pain. The subject examines each picture card and assigns intensity and duration ratings to answer: How does the man feel? (ratings range from 1—no pain, to 7—can't stand pain), and how long will it hurt him? (ranging from 1—not at all, to 7—months). Raw scores are obtained by totalling the ratings for each series. The test can be administered individually or in groups.

INTERPRETATION: Scores for Intensity, Duration, and Intensity + Duration are converted to *T*-scores. Clinical interpretations of Intensity, Duration, and Intensity + Duration of pain are provided for normal male and female adult raw scores, ranging from Very High to Very Low.

RELIABILITY: Split-half reliability coefficients are provided for intensity and duration for each normative sample and range from .56–.89.

VALIDITY: Pain situations were chosen on the basis of a pain survey. Results of validity studies demonstrate consistency in individual pain apperception, neuroticism, and manifest anxiety. Painfulness concepts differed significantly between normal subjects and subjects who are retarded. Picture Cards reflect a high degree of face validity.

SOURCE: Published by: Western Psychological Services, 12031 Wilshire Boulevard, Los Angeles, CA 90025. Tel: 800-648-8857; Fax: 310-478-7838. (**1991**)

COST: $$

SAMPLE: Series II (Anticipation vs. Felt-Sensation)
> 13-A. Man seated in dentist's chair is about to have tooth drilled.
> 13. Same as 13-A, except drill is in man's mouth.

❏ Sensory Integration and Praxis Tests (SIPT)

AUTHOR: A. Jean Ayres

FORMAT: Battery of standardized performance tests.

PURPOSE: SIPT is designed as a diagnostic tool to distinguish between normal children and those with sensory integrative and learning deficits. The tests assess praxis and sensory processing and integration of the vestibular, proprioceptive, tactile, kinesthetic, and visual systems, and thus help in prescribing a course of intervention in these areas.

POPULATION: Children ages 4 years to 8 years, 11 months. (Normative sample consisted of 1,997 children representing a demographic cross-section of the United States.)

SETTING OR POSITION: Quiet, well-lit, distraction-free room, containing child's table and two chairs. Positioning is described for each test.

MATERIALS OR TOOLS: Test manual, scoresheets, and materials are included in the kit; in addition, stopwatch, pencils, paper, and a footstool are needed.

METHOD: The SIPT consists of 17 subtests in the areas of sensory processing, visual–spatial perception, coordination, and motor planning (praxis). Each test includes a list of materials and placement, detailed administration and scoring procedures, and modifications for special circumstances. Tests are generally scored by time, accuracy, and/or successful completion of task. The battery is administered in two sessions if possible, totalling 1-1/2 to 2 hours plus an additional 30–45 minutes for completing protocol sheets for scoring. Individual tests can be administered in about 10 minutes. The protocol sheets are machine processed by the publisher, requiring additional mailing time and scoring fees.

INTERPRETATION: Western Psychological Services performs the computer scoring and can prepare a full-color plotted graph for each subject. Scores compare the subject with the norms and indicate presence (possible or definite) or absence of an impairment. SIPT scores are compared to score profiles typical of various diagnostic groups and help identify the practic or sensory integrative component of learning or behavior problems. Scores should be supplemented by clinical observations and other data about the subject, as well as the administrator's formal training in sensory integration theory and SIPT testing.

RELIABILITY: Test–retest reliability with a 1- or 2-week interval is described as acceptable for most tests or test groups except for four, which showed low test–retest reliability. Interrater reliability between two different raters was high (.94–.99) as were scores on subscales (.85 and above). All users must undergo certification training.

VALIDITY: SIPT demonstrates content validity in the extensive literature search on brain research and consultation with expert faculty members of Sensory Integration International. Concurrent validity is summarized as to how well SIPT differentiates between normal and dysfunctional, as well as between different varieties of dysfunction. There is further evidence of concurrent validity in comparisons of subscale scores with alternate tests (Kaufman, Luria-Nebraska, Bruininks-Oseretsky, Bender-Gestalt, Gessell).

SOURCE: Published by: Western Psychological Services, 12031 Wilshire Boulevard, Los Angeles, CA 90025. Tel: 800-648-8857; Fax: 310-478-7838. (**1989**)

Training and certification through: Sensory Integration International, 1402 Cravens Avenue, Torrance, CA 90501.

COST: $$$$

SAMPLE: Constructional Apraxia

"I'm going to build a house...Here is the floor...Here are the walls...We line up the blocks VERY carefully...Now you build a house like mine here....I'll put the first block here."

❏ Sensory Integration Inventory—Revised, for Individuals with Developmental Disabilities

AUTHORS: Judith E. Reisman, PhD, OTR, FAOTA, and Bonnie Hanschu, OTR

FORMAT: Nonstandardized observation- or interview-based inventory.

PURPOSE: The Inventory is designed to screen individuals with developmental disabilities for possible sensory integrative (SI) dysfunction. It identifies subjects who may benefit from SI treatment and simultaneously screens out those who probably do not have SI dysfunction.

POPULATION: Children and adults with developmentally disabilities and intellectual impairments. It is being tried with other populations who cannot cooperate fully in testing situations (e.g., schizophrenia, Alzheimer's disease).

SETTING OR POSITION: Not specified.

MATERIALS OR TOOLS: User's Guide, Inventory form, pencil.

METHOD: The Inventory consists of four sections associated with sensory integrative processing: tactile, vestibular, proprioceptive, and general reactions. Related items are clustered under subheadings to organize the data. The administrator should be familiar with the subject's typical behavior or interview a parent or caregiver (from home or program staff). Each item is marked yes, no, or unsure of whether the behavior is typical, and whether it has been observed, reported, or elicited in testing. Additional comments are solicited. Duration of the behaviors is noted as long-standing (indicating SI disorder as likely) or recent (another cause likely). User's Guide gives explanatory descriptions of each item. The Inventory can be completed in fewer than 30 minutes.

INTERPRETATION: Items in the Inventory are considered to be "soft signs" as opposed to diagnostic or "hard signs." The interpretation relies on the therapist's judgment to find patterns of dysfunction exhibited by the data. There are no numeric results or cutoff scores.

RELIABILITY: Authors claim there is consistency among raters trained in SI theory. Further studies are in progress.

VALIDITY: Studies in progress.

SOURCE: Available from: PDP Products, 12015 N. July Avenue, Hugo, MN 55038. Tel: 612-439-8865. (**1992**)

SAMPLE: <u>Self-stimulatory behaviors</u>

Y N ? Engages in persistent hand to mouth activity
Mouths objects or clothing

COST: $

❏ Test of Sensory Functions in Infants (TSFI)

AUTHORS: Georgia A. DeGangi, PhD, OTR, and Stanley I. Greenspan, MD

FORMAT: Criterion-referenced rating scale.

PURPOSE: The TSFI, designed as a research or clinical evaluation, is used as a screening tool for sensory integrative dysfunction in infants. In conjunction with other developmental tests, it can help identify infants at risk for learning and emotional disorders.

POPULATION: Infants aged 4–18 months, specifically those with regulatory disorders, developmental delay, and at risk for sensory processing or learning disorders (e.g., high-risk preterm).

SETTING OR POSITION: Infant is seated on parent's lap or on mat or baby blanket with hands, forearms, and feet unclothed.

MATERIALS OR TOOLS: Kit includes manual, scoring sheets, small toys, and stimulus materials.

METHOD: The test consists of 24 items divided into 5 subtests of sensory processing and reactivity: deep pressure, adaptive motor functions, visual-tactile integration, ocular-motor control, and vestibular stimulation. For each item, equipment, administration of the stimulus, and scoring criteria (ranging from adverse—0, to normal—1–3) are described. The test takes about 20 minutes, and is administered individually in one sitting.

INTERPRETATION: Subtest scores provide a profile of the five domains and total test score for the infant's age group. Scores below the cutoff indicate potential problems.

RELIABILITY: Interrater reliability of two observers is .88 to .99. Test–retest reliability varied .26 to .96 depending on domain, with .81 for total test score. The author reports the wide range of coefficients reflects some instability of infant behavior. Reliability of classification scores determined by retesting is .81 to .96.

VALIDITY: Consensus among a panel of experts indicates the items represented the behaviors they were designed to measure, and the subdomains represented the overall domain of sensory functioning. Item discrimination and subtest correlations indicate they measure sufficiently distinct domains. Subtest scores vary in classifying subjects who are normal, delayed, and regulatory disordered; false normal and false delayed error rates are given. Criterion-related validity studies indicate TSFI measures functions distinct from other developmental tests.

SOURCE: Published by: Western Psychological Services, 12031 Wilshire Boulevard, Los Angeles, CA 90025. Tel: 800-648-8857; Fax: 310-478-7838. (**1989**)

COST: $$

SAMPLE: Scoring : 0 = Adverse; 1 = Mild Defensive; 2 = Integrated

Response to Touch: Stomach. Firmly rub the infant's stomach—back and forth—3 times slowly. Repeat once.

Perceptual and Visual–Motor

Assessments

☐ Behavioural Inattention Test (BIT)

AUTHORS: Barbara Wilson, PhD, Janet Cockburn, and Peter Halligan

FORMAT: Standardized battery of behavioral and paper-and-pencil tests.

PURPOSE: The BIT is an instrument for identifying unilateral visual neglect (UVN) and how it affects the subject's daily life. It provides a simple objective and systematic test of everyday skills that reflect capabilities and limitations of visual behavior. The results assist in developing a meaningful rationale for treatment.

POPULATION: Patients suspected of exhibiting UVN due to cerebrovascular accident (CVA), cerebral tumor, or head injury. (Sample consisted of 125 patients admitted to Rivermead Rehabilitation Center in Oxford, England with a presumed unilateral cerebral lesion at average of 2 months following CVA and without complicating factors. Normative data were provided by 50 control subjects from the community who did not suffer from brain damage.)

SETTING OR POSITION: Subject is seated in a quiet room at a table facing the examiner. All test materials are placed in front of the subject's midsagittal plane on a neutral background.

MATERIALS OR TOOLS: Test kit includes manual, scoresheets, scoring template, and stimulus materials (e.g., photographs, telephone number cards). Additional common objects are needed: disconnected telephone, analog clock, short 3-column newspaper article, menu, coins, and playing cards.

METHOD: BIT consists of two components: nine behavioral subtests reflecting aspects of daily life (e.g., telephone dialing, menu reading, coin sorting, map reading) and six conventional pencil-and-paper tasks (e.g., letter cancellations, figure and shape drawing, line bisection). Each subtest includes a brief description, instructions, and scoring directions. Some items can be adapted for dysphasic subjects, and instructions are provided for this purpose. Each subtest is scored by recording the number of omissions; errors of commission are noted but not scored. Cutoff scores for each subtest were set by the control study.

INTERPRETATION: Conventional subtest totals are used to diagnose UVN (as determined by the cutoff score), while behavioral subtest totals are used to construct a profile of the subject's specific strengths and weaknesses in a wide range of visually mediated tasks. Poor scores in the behavior tests alone indicate the need for further perceptual/cognitive evaluation. Observations about the manner in which the subject performs a task should clarify the implications of visual neglect in the subject's everyday life.

RELIABILITY: Interrater reliability of .99 was established by two raters simultaneously scoring each of 13 subjects. A correlation of .91 agreement resulted when parallel forms (two alternative versions of the test) were administered to 10 subjects. Test–retest reliability was .99 with a mean interval of 15 days for 10 subjects.

VALIDITY: Concurrent validity was established by comparing the behavioral subtest scores with the conventional subtest scores for each subject (.92), and the behavioral scores with responses to a short questionnaire filled out by each subject's therapist (.67). Construct and predictive validity are supported by Hartman-Maeir and Katz (1995), who found that most behavioral subtests differentiated between subjects with and without visual neglect, and that scores correlated significantly with similar performance tests and ADL checklists (.63–.89 correlation with 6 of the 9 subtests).

SOURCES: Published by Thames Valley Test Company,

Suffolk, England. Distributed in North America by: National Rehabilitation Services, 117 North Elm Street, PO Box 1247, Gaylord, MI 49735. Tel: 517-732-3866; Fax: 517-732-6164. (**1987**)

Hartman-Maeir, A., & Katz, N. (1995). Validity of the Behavioural Inattention Test (BIT): Relationships with functional tasts. *American Journal of Occupational Therapy, 49*(6), 507–516.

COST: $$$

SAMPLE: Star cancellation

"This page contains stars of different sizes. Look at the page carefully—this is a small star. Every time you see a small star, cross it out like this."

❏ The Chessington O.T. Neurological Assessment Battery (COTNAB)

AUTHORS: Ruth Tyerman, Dip. COT, Andy Tyerman, BA, MSc, Prue Howard, Dip. COT, and Caroline Hadfield, Dip. COT

FORMAT: Standardized battery of performance tests.

PURPOSE: COTNAB was designed to assess functional ability of neurological patients in visual perception, constructional ability, sensorimotor ability, and ability to follow instructions. It is recommended for use as a comprehensive part of an integrated multidisciplinary assessment and treatment program, for initial evaluation, assessing change, and discharge planning.

POPULATION: Adults aged 16–65 with acquired neurological damage. (Standardized on a sample of 150 working-age adults in England, ages 16–65, and 150 patients with primary diagnoses of head injury and stroke.) Initial normative data were collected on the elderly (47 subjects aged 65–87) (Laver & Huchison, 1994).

SETTING OR POSITION: Private room or quiet area with few distractions. The setup of the subject seated at a table with test materials is diagrammed for each subtest.

MATERIALS OR TOOLS: Test kit consists of a large wheeled box containing three notebook files (including Treatment Resource binder), scoring pad, sets of cards, blocks, common objects, dexterity board, and materials for manual construction tasks. In addition, a desk/table, pencil, paper, stop watch, and wire coat hanger are needed. An Introductory Manual and free instructional video are available.

METHOD: COTNAB comprises 12 subtests of eye–hand tasks in the four areas of function listed above. Purpose, design, administration, scoring, and functional implications are described for each subtest. The subject follows verbal instructions and demonstration to perform each timed task. Scores, times, and comments are recorded as each test is completed. Administration requires a minimum of 1 hour and may be spread over 2–3 days. The authors offer recommendations for selecting appropriate subjects and eliminating portions of the tests as needed. Reassessment is suggested after 3 months of treatment and 6 months or more for follow-up.

INTERPRETATION: Ability and Time are combined to give a measure of Overall Performance, since both measures are important to employment prospects. Scoring tables classify times according to age groups (ranging from a++ = Superior, to 0 = Unable/Unwilling to attempt). For each test, scoring tables are used to convert total scores and times to Ability, Time, and Overall Performance grades (ranging from 0, to 5 = Within or above normal limits). The authors offer functional implications of performance in each subtest. Test scores are converted to graph charts for a functional profile of abilities and areas of difficulty. Failure on testing does not necessarily indicate neurological origin; observation of responses, qualitative errors, and awareness of errors should be combined with information from team members in interpreting the nature of impairments. Subtle impairments may not show up on the battery.

RELIABILITY: The authors report highly significant interrater reliability of ability grades; statistics are not given in the Introductory Manual.

VALIDITY: Performance of the head injured and stroke patient samples was compared with performance of the control sample, confirming the value of COTNAB in identifying a wide range of functional impairments. Specific performance differences on each subtest are described for the patient samples, as well as improvement on retesting during the course of rehabilitation.

SOURCES: Published by: Nottingham Rehab Limited,

Nottingham, England . Distributed in the U.S. by: North Coast Medical, 187 Stauffer Blvd., San Jose, CA 95125-1042. Tel: 800-821-9319; Fax 408-283-1950. (**1986**)

Laver, A.J., & Huchison, S. (1994). The performance and experience of normal elderly people on Chessington Occupational Therapy Neurological Assessment Battery (COTNAB). *British Journal of Occupational Therapy, 57*, 137–141.

COST: $$$$

SAMPLE: "In this activity I want you to make a coat hanger.

Using this jig, *(show)* and working from these written instructions *(show)*..."

Developmental Test of Visual-Motor Integration—3rd Revision (VMI)

AUTHORS: Keith E. Beery, and Norman A. Buktenica

FORMAT: Paper-and-pencil graded task performance.

PURPOSE: This test is designed as a classroom screening instrument for early identification of learning difficulties.

POPULATION: Preschool children through adults. (Norms are based on 5,824 children ages 2 years, 9 months through 19 years, 8 months from all major areas of the U.S.; nearly identical norms have been developed for numerous other nationalities.)

SETTING OR POSITION: Subject is seated at a desk with body and test booklet centered and squared with the desk throughout testing.

MATERIALS OR TOOLS: Student Test Booklet, manual, Recording and Scoring sheet, and pencil.

METHOD: The VMI consists of a sequence of 24 geometric forms, graded from simple to complex. A short form of 15 forms may be used for testing children ages 3–8 years. The subject copies each form shown in the space provided in the test booklet. Cues and prompting are permitted. The test may be discontinued after three consecutive forms are failed according to grading criteria. Testing may be done individually (recommended for children under 4 years) or by group in 10–15 minutes. Rater's observations also may be recorded.

INTERPRETATION: Raw score is converted to percentile ranks, standard score for comparison to norms, and age-equivalent scores (used cautiously). The manual briefly discusses remedial teaching related to handwriting skill.

RELIABILITY: Interrater reliability ranged from .58–.99 (median .93 improved to .98 with rater training). Test–retest reliability ranged from .63–.92 (median .81). Split-half reliability ranged from .76 to .91 (median .79).

VALIDITY: Concurrent validity reported in areas of academic skills, chronological age, and with other tests of visual perception and integrative ability. Predictive validity for early academic achievement is noted when used in a battery of prekindergarten tests.

SOURCE: Published by: Modern Curriculum Press, 13900 Prospect Road, Cleveland, OH 44136. Tel: 800-321-3106. (**1967, revised 1982, 1989**)

COST: $ short form; $$ long form

SAMPLE: "The forms are to be copied in order. Only one try on each form is allowed."

❑ Developmental Test of Visual Perception, 2nd Edition (DTVP-2)

AUTHORS: Donald D. Hammill, Nils A. Pearson, and Judith K. Voress

FORMAT: Standardized paper-and-pencil test.

PURPOSE: Derived from Marianne Frostig's test, this second edition is designed to identify disturbances of visual perception and visual-motor integration contributing to learning disabilities. It may be used to determine degree of impairment, need for intervention, and effectiveness of remediation.

POPULATION: Children, ages 4 through 10 years; appropriate for individuals with perceptual impairments, learning disabilities, and physical handicaps; minimum use of language is needed. (Norms are based on 1,972 children from 12 states, representing the U.S. population.)

SETTING OR POSITION: Seated at a table in a well-lit and ventilated private area without distractions.

MATERIALS OR TOOLS: Manual, picture book, response booklets, record forms, and a pencil; computer scoring system is available.

METHOD: The test consists of 8 subtests in which the subject draws, copies, or selects among figures on a page. The subtests are: eye–hand coordination, copying, spatial relationships, position in space, figure–ground, visual closure, visual-motor speed, and form constancy. Each subtest ends when the subject misses a specified number of items. Administration requires 30–60 minutes. Scores are obtained for each subtest (0, 1, or 2 points, generally) and can convert to age equivalents, percentiles, standard scores, and quotients.

INTERPRETATION: Standard scores are graded from Very Poor to Very Superior and allow comparison across subtests, while percentiles compare the subject to the norms. Composite quotients compare visual-perceptual with visual-motor integration ability. Scores can be graphed in profile form to compare scores with each other and for a gross estimate of the subject's strengths and weaknesses.

RELIABILITY: Test–retest reliability over a 2-week interval ranged .71–.86 for subtests, .89 for composites, and .93 for total score. Interrater reliability for all scores was in the .90s. Split-half reliability ranged from means .83–.95 on subtest scores, with all mean composite scores in the .90s.

VALIDITY: The constructs and formats for the test were based on review of the literature and existing tests. Item-discrimination analysis was used to select items. Concurrent validity was supported by high correlation of scores with the Motor-Free Visual Perception Test and the Developmental Test of Visual-Motor Integration. Construct validity studies indicated that DTVP-2 differentiates among ages, that subtests measure different aspects of visual perception, and that scores identify perceptually impaired children. Factor analysis yielded a single factor with loadings by all subtests.

SOURCE: Published by: PRO-ED, Inc., 8700 Shoal Creek Boulevard, Austin, TX 78757. Tel: 512-451-3246; Fax: 800-FXPROED or 800-397-7633. (**1961, revised 1993**)

COST: $$; $ for computer scoring system.

SAMPLE: Position in Space

..."HERE IS A BOX WITH A DRAWING IN IT. OVER HERE ARE THREE OTHER BOXES WITH DRAWINGS IN THEM...LOOK AT THE DRAWING IN THE FIRST BOX. I WANT YOU TO FIND A DRAWING JUST LIKE IT IN ONE OF THESE OTHER BOXES...FIND THE ONE THAT IS IN EXACTLY THE SAME POSITION AS THE FIRST ONE OVER HERE."

❏ Hooper Visual Organization Test (VOT)

AUTHOR: H. Elston Hooper, PhD

FORMAT: Standardized picture identification task.

PURPOSE: This brief and easy-to-administer screening test is intended to measure the ability to integrate visual stimuli. Although it can be used as part of a comprehensive neurological battery, when used alone it appears to be a sensitive indicator of hemispheric damage. It is appropriate for clinical as well as research applications.

POPULATION: Adolescents and adults, 13 years and over; intended for use in a wide variety of settings, including medical, psychiatric, and correctional facilities. Contraindicated if the individual's poor cooperative language ability or thought disorganization impair the ability to respond or understand directions. Cultural bias of the pictures is acknowledged. (Samples consist of junior high and college students, residents in a home for the aged, and an all-male population of a Veterans Administration hospital.)

SETTING OR POSITION: Picture booklet is placed in front of subject.

MATERIALS OR TOOLS: Test manual, booklet of pictures, answer sheet, scoring key, pencil.

METHOD: The test consists of 30 items each containing a simple line drawing of a common object, cut up and rearranged in a puzzle-like manner. The subject is asked to identify the object verbally or in writing. Drawings are graded from simple to complex, requiring fewer than 15 minutes to administer and score. Responses are rated 1 point, 1/2, or 0, according to the scoring key. The test can be administered individually or in groups.

INTERPRETATION: The test yields a Total Raw Score, which can be converted to a corrected raw score to adjust for age and education influences, or a T-score that interprets the probability of impairment (ranging from Very Low to Very High).

RELIABILITY: Studies of split-half reliability on a variety of populations indicate the reliability to be acceptable for clinical use (.78 to .82), according to the author.

VALIDITY: Numerous studies of construct and criterion-related validity are reported, indicating that the VOT scores discriminate among organically impaired, normal, and psychiatric subjects for screening purposes.

SOURCE: Published by: Western Psychological Services, 12031 Wilshire Boulevard, Los Angeles, CA 90025. Tel: 800-648-8857; Fax: 310-478-7838. (**1958, revised 1983**)

COST: $$

SAMPLE: "Look at each cutup picture and decide what it might be if you put it together."

❏ Jordan Left-Right Reversal Test, Third Revised Edition

AUTHOR: Brian T. Jordan, PhD

FORMAT: Norm-referenced paper-and-pencil task with checklists.

PURPOSE: This brief and simple test was designed to assess visual reversals of letters, numbers, and words for early detection and for evaluation of the older student. It can be used in a diagnostic battery for learning disabilities and to recommend remediation.

POPULATION: Students from age 5 years through adulthood. (Norms are based on over 3,000 children, ages 5–12 years, in average classrooms in the Archdiocese school system of New Orleans.) The 12-year-old performance is projected to be equivalent to all older ages.

SETTING OR POSITION: Any classroom or office setting (without visual number or alphabet aids) is adequate; subject is assumed to be seated at a table.

MATERIALS OR TOOLS: Manual, test forms, checklists, paper, and a pencil.

METHOD: The test consists of letter, number, and word reversals at two levels: identification of single letters and numbers for ages 5–8 years, and additional letter reversals within words and word reversals within sentences for ages 9 years and up. The subject marks the reversal; errors are totalled for the score. Individual or group administration requires about 20 minutes. There is an additional laterality checklist to determine hand, eye, ear, foot, and other preferences. Additional material is included for remediation.

INTERPRETATION: Total raw error scores are converted to percentiles with ranges defined for normal, borderline, and deviant performance, the latter associated with neurological learning problems. A deviant score indicates the need for further evaluation. Level I scores are converted to developmental ages with caution. Sex and age (1/2-year increments) norms are given.

RELIABILITY: Test–retest reliability with a 1-week interval showed correlations in the .90s except for the 5-year-old level (.60 with <.01 significance).

VALIDITY: Content validity is based on the selection of symbols and words that present clear reversals when reproduced backwards. Criterion-related validity is based on test scores discriminating between normal and learning disabled children, and on correlations with reading achievement (Wide Range Achievement Test) and perceptual-motor problems (Bender Gestalt Test).

SOURCE: Published by: Academic Therapy Publications, 20 Commercial Blvd., Novato, CA 94947-6191. Tel: 800-422-7249; Fax: 415-883-3720. (**1972, 1980, 1990**)

COST: $

SAMPLE: "On the sheet before you are printed letters and numbers. Some of them are wrong because they are printed backward. Take your pencil and cross out each letter or number that looks backward. ..."

❐ Minnesota Spatial Relations Test (MSRT)

AUTHOR: Rene V. Davis and the University of Minnesota Test Development Division

FORMAT: Standardized performance speed test.

PURPOSE: The test measures speed and accuracy in discriminating and placing three-dimensional geometric shapes in order to assess spatial visualization ability. It was developed for use in assessing industrial and business aptitudes, in employee selection and placement, and for vocational counseling, rehabilitation, and training.

POPULATION: Adolescents and adults. (Norms are based on samples totaling 1,069 individuals from nine educational and industrial groups in four states, generally ages 16 to mid-60s.)

SETTING OR POSITION: Quiet, distraction-free room with adequate ventilation, lighting, and temperature, isolated from other people. Subject stands in front of the table, examiner on the opposite side.

MATERIALS OR TOOLS: Form boards A, B, C, and D, housed in two carrying cases (short form requires two form boards), record form, manual, stopwatch, square table, chair.

METHOD: Approximately 8 minutes are required to administer each pair of form boards. The subject is required to move all of the geometric forms from one form board as rapidly as possible to another in which the spaces are rearranged, and then replace them once again in the first form board. (The short form of the test, though less reliable, stops here.) The task is repeated with the second pair of boards. Only the preferred hand is used.

INTERPRETATION: Two scores are computed: time score and error score, both converted to percentile rank and compared to the appropriate norms.

RELIABILITY: Test–retest and internal consistency studies indicate good reliability generally, though less in short-form error scores. Correlation studies indicate that time and error scores measure separate aspects of spatial visualization ability and may therefore be useful in differentiating the two skill components of speed and accuracy.

VALIDITY: Construct and criterion-related validity are demonstrated in numerous studies, comparing the MSRT with other tests. It has been shown to distinguish among groups expected to have varying levels of spatial relations ability and to predict related job and school performance.

SOURCE: Published by: American Guidance Service, Inc., Publishers Building, Circle Pines, MN 55014. Tel: 800-328-2560; Fax: 612-786-9077. (**1979 revision**)

COST: $$$

SAMPLE: "Remove the blocks from this board, one at a time, and put them into their proper places in this board."

❑ Motor-Free Visual Perception Test-Revised (MVPT-R) and Motor-Free Visual Perception Test-Vertical (MVPT-V)

AUTHORS: Ronald P. Colarusso, EdD, Donald D. Hammill, EdD (MVPT-R), and Louisette Mercier, MA, OTR (MVPT-V)

FORMAT: Standardized nonwritten multiple-choice test.

PURPOSE: The test is designed to provide a quick and simple evaluation of visual perception which avoids motor involvement by the subject. It may be used in screening, diagnosis, and research.

POPULATION: MVPT-R: Children, ages 4 through 11 years, and suitable for a wide range of clinical populations; also applicable for adults. (Revised sample consisted of 912 normal children in Northern California and Georgia.)

MVPT-V: Children and adults with suspected hemifield visual neglect or other visual field cuts; may be used for subjects without visual impairments. (Sample consisted of 39 normal adults and adults with brain-injury, ages 55–79, in Quebec.)

SETTING OR POSITION: Not prescribed. MVPT-V must be placed at midline.

MATERIALS OR TOOLS: MVPT plates, scoring sheet, manual, and pencil.

METHOD: This 40-item, nontimed test assesses visual perception as comprising the following five categories: spatial relationships, visual discrimination, figure–ground, visual closure, and visual memory. The subject is required to point to the correct figure of four alternatives, which matches the stimulus item. The subject is allowed reasonable time (15 seconds is suggested) to respond. Fewer than 10 minutes are required for administration and scoring. Raw scores are converted into perceptual ages (PA) and perceptual quotients (PQ).

MVPT-V consists of 36 stimuli that are arranged vertically instead of horizontally, to eliminate the effect of visual field impairments or neglect.

INTERPRETATION: A PQ of 85 or less is recommended as the criterion for inadequacy on the test, and remediation is indicated. Differences in performance between the MVPT-R and MVPT-V may be due to the presence of visual field impairments that affect scores on the former; new research indicates that scores for individuals with learning disabilities also may be affected due to changes in their saccadic eye movements. For application of the MVPT-R to adults, consult tables for 11-year-olds; mean raw scores remain stable from age 9 and up.

RELIABILITY: For the original version, test–retest (.81 total, ranging .77–.83 for different ages), split-half (.88 total, ranging .81–.84), and inter-item consistency (.86 total, ranging .71–.82) were reported for ages 5 through 8 years, due to small sample of 4-year-olds.

VALIDITY: Content validity is based on literature review of visual perception skill categories. Construct and criterion-related validity are demonstrated by scores increasing with age, correlations of scores with other visual perception tests, and internal consistency via item–test correlations. Finally, test scores were not affected by motor impairments in subjects, confirming its motor-free nature.

SOURCE: Published by: Academic Therapy Publications, 20 Commercial Blvd., Novato, CA 94947-6191. Tel: 800-422-7249; Fax: 415-883-3720. (**1972, revised 1995; Vertical, 1996**)

SAMPLE: "Look at this [stimulus figure]...Find it here...Yes (no), here it is."

COST: $$

❑ OSOT Perceptual Evaluation, Revised (Ontario Society of Occupational Therapists)

AUTHORS: Pat Fisher, Marian Boys, and Claire Holzberg

FORMAT: Performance-based rating scale.

PURPOSE: This clinical assessment was designed to screen for perceptual dysfunction in areas related to basic living skills. It can be used to determine degree of impairment, to monitor change, and to measure effects of treatment and/or spontaneous recovery.

POPULATION: Adults with neurological impairment. (Sample is based on 80 patients of three Toronto Hospitals, aged 42–70, and 70 matched control subjects.)

SETTING OR POSITION: Quiet area with no distractions and test materials within subject's visual range. Subject and examiner are assumed to be seated at a table.

MATERIALS OR TOOLS: Kit includes the manual and test materials (e.g., wire and grommet devices, design cards, blocks, small mannikin, pegboard, formboard, etc.); in addition, stereognosis items, a screen or shield, and pencil are needed.

METHOD: The evaluation consists of 18 items involving brief paper-and-pencil tasks, handling of materials, or simple hand movements. Verbal instructions are provided for each task. Each item is scored according to written criteria from 0 (unable) to 4 (intact), and item scores are totalled. In addition to quantitative measurement, qualitative comments on process and results of task are recorded.

INTERPRETATION: Total scores are rated as follows: 70–72 = Within normal limits, 61–69 = Borderline (requires additional testing), 51–60 = Mild (impairment), 41–50 = Moderate, and 40 or below = Severe.

RELIABILITY: Interrater reliability of two raters scoring 46 subjects was 93.1% agreement on the original version. Internal consistency for the 18 test items was .90.

VALIDITY: Comparisons of scores between patient and normal samples indicated that score totals differentiated between the two groups, as well as among degrees of impairment (mild, moderate, severe). The instrument was sufficiently sensitive to establish cutoff scores (70 and above is nonimpaired and 60 and below is impaired) with 100% probability. There is no discussion of the relationship of these tabletop tasks to basic living skills.

SOURCE: Published by: Nelson Canada (sister company NFER-NELSON), 1120 Birchmount Road, Scarborough, Ontario M1K 5G4, Canada. Tel: 800-268-2222; Fax: 416-752-9646. (**1991**)

COST: $$$$

SAMPLE: SCANNING

> "Can you read these letters?"
> "Cross out all the H's you find on this sheet, like this." Demonstrate by crossing out the first "H" on the (L) side of the top line.

❑ Rivermead Perceptual Assessment Battery (RPAB)

AUTHORS: Gita Bhavnani, Janet Cockburn, Nadina Lincoln, and Susan Whiting

FORMAT: Standardized battery of performance tasks.

PURPOSE: These easy-to-administer tasks are designed for use by occupational therapists to assess visual-perceptual dysfunction following a stroke or head injury. The battery can be used as an initial assessment and to monitor progress over time.

POPULATION: Adults, ages 16–97 years. (Normative sample consisted of 69 normal adults, ages 16–69 years, from the hospital staff and community of Rivermead Rehabilitation Centre in England.)

SETTING OR POSITION: Examiner is seated adjacent or at a right angle to the preferred or unaffected side of the subject.

MATERIALS OR TOOLS: Test kit consists of a carrying case with manual, record forms, layout guide, and subtest materials: picture cards, test sheets, common objects (e.g., cup, comb), wooden body parts, cubes, and geometrical shapes.

METHOD: The battery comprises 16 short tasks that assess form and color constancy, sequencing, object completion, figure–ground discrimination, body image, inattention, and spatial awareness. Standardized instructions are given for each subtest, and the required materials are placed on the layout guide, which serves as a uniform background for the tasks. There is a 3- to 5-minute time limit for 15 of the subtests; total administration time is 45–60 minutes. (Shortened versions of the battery have been studied by Lincoln and Edmans [1989].) Scoring instructions for each subtest (e.g., 1 point given for each correct response) are described in the manual and recorded on the record form.

INTERPRETATION: Scores are summarized and plotted on a graph to represent extent and pattern of impairment. They are interpreted using the normative tables according to three different intelligence levels. Because intelligence was found to influence scores, premorbid intelligence level of the subject must be estimated (above average, average, or below average) using one of three recommended vocabulary tests or by other subjective means. The type and extent of deficit are determined by the number of subtest scores falling below the expected scores and by the discrepancy between actual and expected scores.

RELIABILITY: Test–retest reliability for left hemiplegic adults o1 year post–right hemisphere stroke, with a 4-week interval between testing, exhibited reliability for 11 tests; 5 remaining tests were revised and retested. Interrater reliability on videotaped assessments exhibited significant agreement on all tests (.89–1.00 on all but two subtests) with perfect agreement on three subtests.

VALIDITY: Most subtests correlate well with other psychological tests known to be good measures of visual perception. Test scores discriminate between normal and brain-damaged adults, and between normal and right cerebrovascular (CVA) patients.

SOURCES: Published by: NFER-NELSON Publishing Company Ltd. Distributed in the U.S. by: Western Psychological Services, 12031 Wilshire Boulevard, Los Angeles, CA 90025-1251. Tel: 800-648-8857; Fax: 310-478-7838. (**1985**)

Laver, A.J. (1990). Test reviews: Rivermead Perceptual Assessment Battery (RPAB). In J.R. Beech, & L. Harding, (Eds.), *Assessment of the Elderly*. Windsor, England: NFER-Nelson.

Lincoln, N.B., & Edmans, J. A. (1989). A shortened

version of the Rivermead Perceptual Assessment Battery. *Clinical Rehabilitation, 3,* 215–221.

COST: $$$$

SAMPLE: Object Matching

Place the objects in order over the layout guide as shown...

Pick up and show two yellow cups. Then place them together at the base of the board. Say:

Now you go on.

☐ Test of Visual-Motor Skills (TVMS) and Test of Visual-Motor Skills: Upper Level Adolescents and Adults (TVMS:UL)

AUTHOR: Morrison F. Gardner

FORMAT: Standardized paper-and-pencil task.

PURPOSE: This test is designed as a precise and accurate method for assessing how a child or adult visually perceives nonlanguage forms and translates what is perceived through hand function (i.e., by eye–hand coordination). It is intended for clinical use and as an aid in planning remediation.

POPULATION: Children from 2 to 13 years of age. (Sample consisted of 1,009 normal children from preschool programs through seventh grade in the San Francisco Bay area.)

UL: adolescents and adults from ages 12–40 years. (Sample consisted of 878 students in the Bay area.)

SETTING OR POSITION: A warm, friendly, pleasant environment with good lighting, no visual or auditory distractions, and a desk and chair for the subject.

MATERIALS OR TOOLS: Test booklet and manual, pencil.

METHOD: The TVMS consists of 26 geometric forms or designs (or 16 in UL) graded in difficulty, each on a single plate with ample room for copying. The subject is asked to draw each form in the booklet, from beginning to end or until four consecutive failures. Each form is scored 0 (unable to copy), 1 (errors present), or 2 (successfully completed). Criteria and samples are provided to assist in scoring judgments. In addition, the examiner is to record subject's test behavior and to note drawing characteristics for diagnostic purposes. Test administration takes 5–20 minutes and can be conducted individually or in groups.

INTERPRETATION: The test yields a total score, which is converted to motor age, standard score, and percentile rank according to the norms. Examination of the pattern of errors offer clinical and diagnostic information to suggest remediation.

RELIABILITY: Split-half reliability ranged from .31 to .90 with a median value of .82; all but the lowest coefficient were within acceptable range according to the author. UL: split-half reliability across all age levels was .86.

VALIDITY: Content validity is based on item reviews by experts in psychology and testing. Criterion-related validity is demonstrated by item-by-item correlations with the Developmental Test of Visual-Motor Integration (VMI) and total score correlations with VMI (.92; UL .46–.64) and the Bender Visual Motor Gestalt Test (.75; UL .31–.80), as well as other tests summarized in the manual. TVMS exhibited a correlation of .69 with the TVMS:UL for the overlapping 12-year-old sample.

SOURCE: Published by: Psychological and Educational Publications, Inc., 1477 Rollins Road, Burlingame, CA 94010. Tel: 800-523-5775; Fax: 800-447-0907. (**1986; UL 1993**)

COST: $; UL $$.

SAMPLE: "I want you to copy with your pencil some designs or forms. Now turn your page to the first form, which is a circle."

❐ Test of Visual-Perceptual Skills (Non-Motor) (TVPS) and Test of Visual-Perceptual Skills (Non-Motor): Upper Level (TVPS:UL)

AUTHOR: Morrison F. Gardner

FORMAT: Standardized multiple-choice test (nonwritten).

PURPOSE: This test is designed to determine a child's visual–perceptual strengths and weaknesses without the use of motor responses. It is intended for clinical use and to aid in planning remediation. It can help in distinguishing between visual-perceptual impairment and motoric dysfunction.

POPULATION: Children from 4 through 12 years of age. (Sample consisted of 1,200 preschool- and school-aged children of normal functioning from the San Francisco Bay area, selected to represent the range and level of ability of the U.S. population for each age.)

UL: adolescents ages 12–18 years of age. (Sample consisted of 664 students representative of U.S. racial and ethnic makeup.)

SETTING OR POSITION: Pleasant, well-illuminated environment, free from distractions, noise or interruptions.

MATERIALS OR TOOLS: Manual, Individual Record Form, pencil.

METHOD: Each of seven factors is assessed by means of 16 items arranged progressively according to difficulty for each subtest. The seven subtests are: visual discrimination, visual memory, visual–spatial relations, visual form constancy, visual sequential memory, visual figure–ground, and visual closure. The test item is shown and subject indicates the correct choice among the response pictures on the test plate. The subject's responses are recorded, as is test behavior (e.g., distractibility, cooperation). Raw scores are calculated for each subtest to yield a total score. The test is administered individually in approximately 10–20 minutes and can be used with language-impaired and physically disabled subjects.

INTERPRETATION: Raw scores are converted to perceptual ages, standard scores, and percentile ranks compared to the normal distribution. Low functioning in the tested areas suggest possible difficulty in learning. Performance across subtests determine relative strengths and weaknesses in visual perception.

RELIABILITY: TVPS: internal consistency is demonstrated for each subtest (median coefficients range from .66 to .80) and for the total score (median .90), although some subtest coefficients for the older age ranges are noted to be low.

UL: coefficients range from .25–.52, with improved reliability if projections are made to a larger number of test items.

VALIDITY: Evidence of content, criterion-related, and possible predictive validity are summarized. They are based generally on literature review to identify the seven factors of visual perception; item correlations with subtest and total scores and rank-ordering of items by difficulty; discrimination of scores between normal and learning-impaired groups; correlation of scores with other tests that tap visual–perceptual skills; and low correlations of scores between TVPS and reading and spelling subtests of the Wide Range Achievement Test.

SOURCE: Published by: Psychological and Educational Publications, Inc., 1477 Rollins Road, Burlingame, CA 94010. Tel: 800-523-5775; Fax: 800-447-0907. (**1982; UL 1993**)

COST: $$

SAMPLE: "Look at this form . . . find it among the five forms below."

Infant and Child Development

(Neuromusculoskeletal/Developmental)

Assessments

☐ Assessment of Preterm Infants' Behavior (APIB)

AUTHORS: Heidelise Als, PhD, Barry M. Lester, PhD, Edward Z. Tronick, PhD, and T. Berry Brazelton, MD

FORMAT: Behavior checklist and scale.

PURPOSE: This comprehensive assessment provides a neurodevelopmental diagnostic instrument for neonatal specialists. It is designed to document patterns of the infant's developing behavioral organization.

POPULATION: Prematurely born infants who can be handled in room temperature and room air without medical or technological aids. (Sample of 38 preterm infants at Children's Hospital, Boston were assigned to the experimental study in the reference below.)

SETTING OR POSITION: A semi-lighted quiet environment is recommended.

MATERIALS OR TOOLS: Manual, scoring booklet, and pencil; in addition, stimulation materials consist of flashlight, gentle red rattle, orange stick, red ball.

METHOD: APIB consists of six packages of increasingly demanding environmental stimulation: sleep/distal, uncover/supine, low tactile, medium tactile/vestibular, high tactile/vestibular, and attention/interaction. Each package assesses function and integration of five systems: physiological, motor, state, attentional/interactive, and regulatory. Maneuvers consisting of external stimuli (light, rattle) or handling are administered in sequence and scored according to directions for each item. Many items are scored based on appearance and behavior overall (e.g., skin color, robustness, and endurance). Each package yields three scores for each system: baseline (state of organization prior to administering maneuvers), reaction (degree of reactivity and relative disorganization of a system during administration of maneuvers), and postpackage (state of organiza-

tion following maneuvers reflecting infant's regulatory ability). Scores range from 1 (little or none of the behavior) to 9 (a lot of a behavior). An additional examiner facilitation score reflects the degree of aid needed from the examiner to optimize the infant's performance or stability. Two supplemental sheets contain a 4-point scale for eye movements and a rating form for asymmetry of performance.

INTERPRETATION: Scores are transferred to a System Organization Graph that illustrates the infant's behavior in each system across the six packages. Results are useful in determining diagnosis, planning intervention, determining follow-up, and serving as an outcome measure.

RELIABILITY: Education and training sessions are conducted to ensure reliability of the examiner's administration, observation, and scoring skills.

VALIDITY: APIB is based on the Synactive Theory of Development by Dr. Als and is an extension and adaptation of the Brazelton Neonatal Behavioral Assessment Scale. (For more information, see Newborn Individualized Developmental Care and Assessment Program elsewhere in this text.) APIB scores were significantly higher when used as the neurodevelopmental outcome measure for preterm infants given individualized developmental care in a neonatal intensive care unit; they correlated with medical and electrophysiological outcome measures and with behavioral outcomes using Bayley Scales of Infant Development. There is further evidence of predictive ability to neuropsychological function and school achievement at ages 5 and 8 years.

SOURCES: Materials and training information available through the author at: Neurobehavioral Infant and Child Studies, Children's Hospital, 300 Longwood

Avenue, Boston, MA 02115. Tel: 617-355-6179; Fax: 617-355-7230; e-mail: love@al.tch.harvard.edu (contact: Geoffrey Love). **(1979)**

Als, H., Lawhon, G., Duffy, F.H., McAnulty, G.B., Gibes-Grossman, R., Blickman, J.G. (1994). Individualized developmental care for the very low-birth-weight preterm infant: Medical and neurofunctional effects. *Journal of the American Medical Association, 272,* 853–858.

Fleisher, B.E., VandenBerg, K., Constantinou, J., Heller, C., Benitz, W.E., Johnson, A., Rosenthal, A., Stevenson, D.K. (1995). Individualized developmental care for very-low-birth-weight premature infants. *Clinical Pediatrics, 34*(10): 523–529.

COST: $$$ for training and materials; $$$ for follow-up reliability session.

SAMPLE: Package I: Sleep/distal
LIGHT
Timing of Response
1. All responses instantaneous with *onset* of stimulus. ...
4. Considerable delay of some responses.
9. Responses in modulated interval from onset of stimulus. ...

❑ Bayley Infant Neurodevelopmental Screener (BINS)

AUTHOR: Glen P. Aylward

FORMAT: Checklist based on observation of behavior.

PURPOSE: BINS is designed to identify infants with neurological impairment or developmental delay. As a screening test, it indicates the need for further assessment.

POPULATION: Infants ages 3–24 months. (Standardization sample is based on a normal sample of 100 infants at each of 6 ages and representative of the U.S. population; and a clinical sample of 303 infants from neonatal intensive care unit follow-up clinics or previously diagnosed as developmentally delayed.)

SETTING OR POSITION: Distraction-free environment with primary caregiver present; mat or blanket on tabletop for infants under 1 year, chair and table, and stairs for older infants; positioning is described for each item.

MATERIALS OR TOOLS: Kit contains manual, record forms, stimulus cards, and manipulable objects in a carrying case; additional paper and pencil are needed.

METHOD: BINS consists of six item sets for different developmental ages. Each set contains 11–13 items that assess four areas of abilities: Basic Neurological Functions, auditory and visual Receptive Functions, verbal and motor Expressive Functions, and Cognitive Processes. BINS includes items from the Bayley Scales of Infant Development, 2nd edition, but scored to assess quality as well as presence of movement. Instructions for each item include position, materials, administration (presentation of stimuli and observation of resulting behavior), and scoring criteria. Items are scored as optimal (1) or nonoptimal (0); optimal items are summed for a total score. Administration requires 10 minutes.

INTERPRETATION: Cutoff scores distinguish among infants with low, moderate, and high risk of impairment, and assist in determining type of dysfunction: global (across the four areas of function) or specific, and static (without further deterioration) or progressive. Isolated pathologic indicators (e.g., hypotonia, abnormal eye movements) may be observed during testing and should be evaluated further.

RELIABILITY: Test–retest reliability with an interval of less than a week ranges from .71–.84 across ages. Interrater reliability between administrator and observer ranges from .79–.96. Internal consistency reliability ranges from. 73–.85.

VALIDITY: Varying agreement between BINS cut scores and results of other developmental measures (Bayley Scales of Infant Development-Second Edition, Battelle Developmental Inventory, and Denver II) is discussed.

SOURCE: Published by: The Psychological Corporation, 555 Academic Court, San Antonio, TX 78204-2498. Tel: 800-228-0752; Fax: 800-232-1223. (**1995**)

COST: $$$

SAMPLE: Raises Self to Standing Position

Administration Lie the infant on the floor close to a chair. "Shake the bell and then place it on the edge of the chair.

Scoring Score the infant's performance as 1(optimal) if she raises herself to a standing position, using a chair or other convenient object for support.

Score the performance as 0 (nonoptimal) if the infant does not raise herself to a standing position.

❏ Bayley Scales of Infant Development, 2nd Edition (BSID-II)

AUTHOR: Nancy Bayley

FORMAT: Standardized rating scale based on observation of behavior.

PURPOSE: The scales are designed to provide a tripartite (mental, motor, and social/object relationships) evaluation of the child's early developmental status. It is used to diagnose developmental delay and plan intervention strategies, follow progress after intervention, and as a research tool.

POPULATION: Children ages 1–42 months. (Norms are based on a national, stratified random sample of 1,700 normal children representing the U.S. population.)

SETTING OR POSITION: Large, quiet, well-lit examining room free of distraction, with a padded surface or child-size table and chairs, depending on the age of the subject. Stairs may be needed. Subject's starting position is given for each item.

MATERIALS OR TOOLS: Test kit includes the manual, stimulus booklet and cards, record forms, and all necessary materials except for paper, tissues, plastic bags, and a stopwatch.

METHOD: The instrument consists of three parts: the Mental Scale (178 items), the Motor Scale (111 items), and the Behavior Rating Scale (30 items). Mental and Motor Scales assess current level of development in four facets: language, cognitive, personal–social, and fine and gross motor. The Behavior Rating Scale (BRS) assesses the child's test behavior (e.g., attention, engagement, quality of movement), with background information from the caregiver. With caregiver present, the examiner establishes rapport with the child and proceeds with age-appropriate test items. Test stimuli designed to engage the child are presented and the child's responses are graded (credit/no credit for Mental and Motor Scales

and 5-point scale for BRS); specific intructions for administration, timing, and scoring criteria are given for each item. Sequence of items is flexible, and the test may take from 25–60 minutes. Testing a child with a disability is discussed briefly in the manual.

INTERPRETATION: The test yields a Mental Development Index (MDI) and Psychomotor Development Index (PDI) based on comparison with the normative population; a profile of developmental age scores across the four facets can be charted to show the child's level of functioning and relative strengths and weaknesses. Cutoff scores for BRS indicate within normal limits, questionable, or nonoptimal results; interpretations are discussed for the total score, factor scales, item analysis, and comparison with MDI and PDI.

RELIABILITY: Reliability coefficients average .88 for Mental Scale, .84 for Motor Scale, and .88 for total BRS score (ranging .74–.88 for facet averages). Interrater reliability between examiner and observor is .96 (Mental), .75 (Motor, only examiner manipulating child), and adequate for the more subjective BRS, as determined by various studies. Test–retest reliability with 1- to16-day interval has mean agreement of .87 (Mental) and .78 (Motor) for all ages, and .60–.71 for facets of the BRS at ages 24 and 36 months; improvement in scores may reflect maturation and practice.

VALIDITY: Content analysis involved item review by experienced BSID users and child development experts and subsequent revision to ensure correct classification and absence of bias (gender, race, culture). Construct validity is supported by the literature as well as correlation studies showing that scales are distinct constructs that correlate with total scores; in addition, factor analysis was used to classify items according to the facets. BSID-II correlations with BSID (the original), McCarthy Scales of Children's Abilities, Wechsler

Preschool and Primary Scale of Intelligence, and others are reviewed. Comparisons of normative sample to special populations of high-risk children are discussed, and predictive validity (to later development and IQ) of the original BSID is summarized.

SOURCE: Published by: The Psychological Corporation, 555 Academic Court, San Antonio, TX 78204-2498. Tel: 800-228-0752; Fax: 800-232-1223. **(1969, revised 1993)**

COST: $$$$; purchase restricted to qualified users.

SAMPLE: Mental Scale
        Inspects Own Hand(s)
        Smiles at Mirror Image

Behavior Rating Instrument for Autistic and Other Atypical Children, 2nd Edition (BRIAAC)

AUTHORS: Bertram A. Ruttenberg, MD, Enid G. Wolf-Schein, EdD, CCC-SLP, and Charles Wenar, PhD

FORMAT: Observation-based rating scales.

PURPOSE: This set of behavior scales is designed to evaluate, by direct observation, the present functional status and behavior changes in an otherwise "untestable" population. It offiers a comprehensive picture of behavior in a developmental context. It is intended for therapeutic and educational program planning and research.

POPULATION: Children exhibiting autism, severely developmentally delayed deafness and/or blindness, or other severe emotional disturbances of early onset (before age 3). The scales measure behaviors equivalent to the developmental range from birth to 3.5–4.5 years of age (depending on the scale). Preliminary studies suggest that BRIAAC can be used with low-functioning adults.

SETTING OR POSITION: Subject's usual environment.

MATERIALS OR TOOLS: Kit consists of the manual and report form master sheets (with permission to reproduce them); and a pencil.

METHOD: BRIAAC assesses 7 areas of function characteristically affected in atypical children: relationship to adult, communication, drive for mastery, vocalization and expressive speech, sound and speech reception, social responsiveness, and psychobiological development (The body movement scale is available only in the first edition for those especially interested in this area.) Two supplementary scales, expressive and receptive gesture and sign language, assess those who use nonvocal communication. Each scale consists of 10 levels of behavior progressing from most disturbed to that of a normal 3- to 4-year-old. The rater observes a sample of the child's activities for a minimum of 2 hours in a variety of the child's typical settings. Following the completion of observation, the rater scores observed behaviors on all 7 scales by distributing a total of 10 points among the levels of each scale. As an alternative, scoring may be done by checklist, identifying behaviors as frequent, occasional, or not observed, and based on observation or interview with someone familiar with the child. Scales can be administered individually or in total. Scale scores range from 10 (most disturbed) to 100 (adequate function). Supplementary and qualitative information is recorded separately. Training is strongly recommended for raters; certification is available for reliability training.

INTERPRETATION: Ratings result in a behavioral profile useful in clinical assessment, planning remediation, and research. The scale scores can be charted on an interscale profile as a visual representation of results; they also can be totalled for a cumulative score to compare degree of disturbance among children or to evaluate change. BRIAAC can be used to develop Individualized Education Programs, for therapy recommendations, and for research.

RELIABIITY: Interrater reliability ranging from .84 to .93 on scale scores was demonstrated by pairs of raters. Test–retest reliability ranged from .61 to .91 on scale scores over a 2- to 3-week interval.

VALIDITY: Content validity is demonstrated by extensive review and revision of items by experts in many fields of health and education. Concurrent validity is supported in several studies by correlation of scores with expert clinicians' rankings (ranges of .43–.83 and .57–94 with scale scores; .95 with cumulative score). The order of levels within scales is supported by data analysis of subject scores. Factor analysis supports a common complex factor characterized as "reality participation."

BRIAAC scores differentiate between the target population and other groups of children. Numerous other studies are described supporting the value of the BRIAAC with a variety of populations and its uses in research.

SOURCES: Published by: Stoelting Co., 620 Wheat Lane, Wood Dale, IL 60191. Tel: 800-860-9775; Fax: 708-860-9775. (**1977, 1991**)

For training workshops, contact: Enid G. Wolf-Schein, EdD, CCC-SLP, 1703 Andros Isle, Suite J-2, Coconut Creek, FL 33066.

COST: $$

SAMPLE: Relationship to an Adult Scale

1. Impervious or oblivious to the presence of another person.
2. Withdrawal or intermittent fleeting responses. "Tuning in and out."

❏ Callier-Azusa Scale

AUTHORS: Robert Stillman, PhD (editor of G edition); H Scale: Robert Stillman, PhD and Christy Battle, MS

FORMAT: Observation-based behavioral scale.

PURPOSE: This developmental scale was designed to assess severely handicapped children, particularly at lower developmental levels in the classroom. It may be used to recommend the developmental level appropriate for activity selection and to evaluate developmental progress.

POPULATION: Deaf–blind and severely and profoundly handicapped children. (Research samples for reliability and validity studies are briefly described.)

SETTING OR POSITION: G scale requires observation of behaviors typically occurring in classroom activities. H scale requires observation in a variety of physical and interpersonal contexts.

MATERIALS OR TOOLS: Scale manual (original G scale or H scale) and scoresheet, pencil; any other materials needed are commonly found in the everyday environment.

METHOD: The G scale consists of 18 subscales in 5 areas: motor development; perceptual development; daily living skills; cognition, communication, and language; and social development. Each area includes behaviors that make up developmental milestones and are common to classroom activities. Individuals very familiar with the child's behavior (e.g., teachers, parents) observe the subject over a 2-week period. They rate the items according to general criteria as to whether the behaviors are well integrated (i.e., occur spontaneously and are appropriately generalized).

The H scale was designed for use by professionals to assess communication in four developmental domains: representational and sumbolic abilities, receptive communication, intentional communication, and reciprocity. Each domain consists of sequential steps or milestones and are rated as above.

INTERPRETATION: The test scores yield a profile of development inthe five areas. Age equivalencies for each item based on normal development are printed on the profile sheet. The importance of the scale is the sequence in which the behaviors occur and not the age norms.

RELIABILITY: Interrater reliability for groups of four individual observers and between teams of two observers ranged from .66 –.97, lowest in the area of social development, as expected. Agreement among subitems is high (90% socialization, 92% tactile).

VALIDITY: Since no standard population exists, sequential validity of items was examined, yielding scaleability coefficients well above the acceptable level of .6 to indicate the scale is ordinal.

SOURCE: Obtain test materials and research reprints from the author at: University of Texas at Dallas, Callier Center for Communication Disorders, 1966 Inwood Road, Dallas, TX 75235. Tel: 214-883-3060 (or author: -3106); Fax: 214-883-3006. (**G edition, 1978; H scale addendum, 1984**)

COST: $

SAMPLE: Visual development:

(A) Attempts to secure object beyond his reach.
(B) Turns objects in his hand and explores them visually.

❒ Clinical Observations of Motor and Postural Skills (COMPS)

AUTHORS: Brenda N. Wilson, MS, OT(C), Nancy Pollock, MSc, OT(C), Bonnie J. Kaplan, PhD, and Mary Law, PhD, OT(C)

FORMAT: Performance-based screening test.

PURPOSE: This standardization of traditional clinical observations used by pediatric occupational therapists serves as a screening tool for the identification of motor problems with a postural component in children.

POPULATION: Children, ages 5–9 years, without known neurological or neuromotor problems or general intellectual delays. (Sample consisted of 67 children who demonstrated developmental coordination disorder [DCD], and 56 children with no known motor problems.)

SETTING OR POSITION: Quiet 8' x 10' room with minimal distractions. For each item, position of the subject is described as either seated or on the floor (supine, quadruped, prone).

MATERIALS OR TOOLS: Carrying portfolio that contains manual, two measurement tools, and scoresheets; in addition, chairs, mat, stopwatch, and a pencil are needed.

METHOD: COMPS consists of six items: slow movements, rapid forearm rotation, finger–nose touching, prone extension posture, asymmetrical tonic neck reflex, and supine flexion posture. For each item, a simple motor task is described and demonstrated by the examiner, after which the subject performs it. Scoring criteria vary and are described with each item. Scores are totalled, including duration and quality scores, converted to weighted scores, and adjusted for age of the subject. COMPS can be administered in 15–20 minutes, individually or in groups, and is easy to learn and score.

INTERPRETATION: Scores of less than zero indicate problems in postural and motor skills and the need for further assessment; scores of more than zero indicate normal functioning. (COMPS weighted scores for the different age groups are based on a small population sample and do not represent norms.) Item scores may indicate specific dysfunction, and the authors guide individual item interpretations.

RELIABILITY: Test–retest reliability within a 2-week interval for both groups and the total sample was significant (DCD=.87, non-DCD=.76, total=.93). Interrater reliability for four raters of varying levels of experience was statistically significant but varied with the subject groups and levels of experience. Internal consistency was acceptable for the total test (. 77 with item total correlates ranging from .33-.53).

VALIDITY: Total scores for DCD and non-DCD groups differed significantly at each age level and in the total sample; most items discriminated strongly between the two groups. The test's senstivity to detection of dysfunction was 82% and 100% for the different age groups; its specificity in identifying children without motor problems ranged from 63–90%. The authors summarize concurrent validity correlations with numerous other measures, finding that postural items related to other tests of balance and vestibular-related functions.

SOURCE: Published by: Therapy Skill Builders, a division of Psychological Corporation, 555 Academic Court, San Antonio, TX 78204-2498. Tel: 800-228-0752; Fax: 800-232-1223. (**1994**)

COST: $

SAMPLE: Prone Extension Posture

"I am going to fly like Superman (or Supergirl). See how I raise everything off the floor at the same time? Then I hold it as long as I can. Now you try it."

❐ Denver II

AUTHORS: William K. Frankenburg, MD, MSPH, Josiah Dodds, PhD, Philip Archer, ScD, Beverly Bresnick, MA, Patrick Maschka, MA, Norma Edelman, and Howard Shapiro, PhD

FORMAT: Standardized task performance and observation screening tool.

PURPOSE: The tool was designed to provide a simple method for early identification of children at risk for developmental problems. It gives a brief overview of the child's development.

POPULATION: Children, ages 1 month to 6 years. (Norms are based on a quota sample of over 2,000 children from Denver County and 20 other Colorado counties.)

SETTING OR POSITION: Parent may hold child; specific positioning described as needed for each item.

MATERIALS OR TOOLS: Training and technical (optional) manuals, scoresheet, test kit containing 11 small manipulatives and toys in a zippered bag, and a pencil; a table and chair are needed for some test items.

METHOD: The test consists of 125 items in four areas: personal–social, fine motor–adaptive, language, and gross motor. After calculating the child's age onto the scoresheet, the examiner administers items below the subject's age level (or within capabilities) and advances until the child fails three items. Each item is arranged chronologically on the chart by the age of the child and marked pass/fail. Test behavior during administration is marked on a checklist (compliance, interest in surroundings, etc.). Items not observed can be scored by caregiver report. Item scores are correlated with chronological age to identify age-appropriate versus delayed behaviors. Administration requires about 20 minutes; examiner training is recommended by the publisher.

Related materials are available: Prescreening Developmental Questionnaire for parents, Home Screening Questionnaire to assess the home environment, and more. An abbreviated version of the test is in process.

INTERPRETATION: Item scores correlated with chronological age level yield an interpretation of normal, abnormal, questionable, or untestable. Results from one testing should be interpreted with caution, and ongoing surveillance of the child is recommended. The screening test is one factor in the context of the larger picture of the child; the examiner is referred to the technical manual for subgroup and composite norms and for influencing factors. Denver II is not a predictive or diagnostic instrument.

RELIABILITY: Interrater reliability among raters trained to obtain < 90% reliability demonstrated excellent reliability between examiner and observer, averaging .99. Test–retest reliability over a 7- to 10-day interval averaged .90.

VALIDITY: High degree of face validity is exhibited by the age placement of individual items and the precision with which passing scores corresponded with age during the standardization process. The test interpretation categories and referral criteria (normal, abnormal, etc.) were based on clinical judgment and await further study. (Agreement with Stanford-Binet and Baylet was established for the original version [1967].)

SOURCES: Published by: Denver Developmental Materials, Inc. (1967, 1975, 1989), PO Box 6919, Denver, CO 80206. Tel: 800-419-4729.

Frankenburg, W.K., Dodds, J., Archer, P., Shapiro, H., & Bresnick, B. (1992). The Denver II: A major revision and restandardization of the Denver Developmental Screening Test. *Pediatrics, 89*(1), 91–96.

Frankenburg, W., & Dodds, J. (1967). The Denver

Development Screening Test. *Journal of Pediatrics, 71*(2), 181–191.

SAMPLE: PERSONAL–SOCIAL

> Smile spontaneously
> Smile responsively
> Regard own hand

COST: $$; training video $$$ (rental $$).

❑ Developmental Programming for Infants and Young Children

AUTHORS: Edited by D. Sue Schafer and Martha S. Moersch (vols. 1-3), and by Diane B. D'Eugenio and Martha S. Moersch (vols. 4-5)

FORMAT: Developmental checklist.

PURPOSE: The program is intended to combine assessment with treatment planning and implementation in a wide range of functions. Meant for use by an interdisciplinary team, it provides a systematic evaluation of development for the purpose of designing an individualized curriculum. It is best used as a supplement to standard testing.

POPULATION: Children functioning in the 0- to 60-month developmental age range (0–36 months in volumes 1–3 and 3- to 5-year-olds in volumes 4 and 5), including normal, high-risk, and handicapped populations. (Field test for 3- to 5-year-olds was completed on 71 preschool children at 4 sites, in addition to 92 children from Missouri daycare centers who participated in field testing of the cognition section. Infant norms were derived from the original item sources.)

SETTING OR POSITION: Small, comfortable, quiet, room, free of other stimulating materials if possible.

MATERIALS OR TOOLS: Developmental Profile programs, which contain a list of common objects and materials required. For nonambulatory children, a mat is needed in addition to a chair and table for parent or ambulatory child.

METHOD: The program contains two separate evaluations: the Early Intervention Developmental Profile (vol. 2) and instructions (vol. 1), and the Preschool Development Profile (vol. 5) and instructions (vol. 4). (Volume 3 contains program suggestions for the younger age group.) The Profiles both consist of six scales: perceptual/fine motor, cognition, language, social/emotional, self-care, and gross motor development. Each contains over 200 items and can be administered in an hour. An interdisciplinary team begins by observing the child to estimate the appropriate level of development for testing. Each item is scored "pass" or "fail," according to standard instructions and criteria. The highest level achieved in each area is plotted on the Profile Graph.

INTERPRETATION: The evaluation yields a profile of current developmental age levels with areas of relative strength and weakness.

RELIABILITY: Interrater reliability exhibited a mean of .89 agreement, and test–retest ranged from .90 to .98 correlation for the Early Profile.

VALIDITY: Concurrent validity was established by correlating the scales with other standardized tests during item selection. Original items are based on current developmental theories and were scrutinized by experts in each area.

SOURCE: Published by: University of Michigan Press (1977, revised 1981), 389 Greene Street, Ann Arbor, MI 48104. Tel: 313-764-4394; Fax: 313-936-0456.

SAMPLE: Social–emotional (28–31 months)

Identifies self in mirror: Show the child his/her image in a mirror. Ask who that is. Pass if the child gives his/her own name.

COST: $

❐ Erhardt Developmental Prehension Assessment (EDPA) (Revised) and Short Screening Form (EDPA-S)

AUTHOR: Rhoda Priest Erhardt, MS, OTR

FORMAT: Checklist based on observation and task performance.

PURPOSE: The EDPA was designed to chart prehensile development and describe hand skills of the delayed and/or abnormal child, although it can also be used to chart normal prehension as well. EDPA-S can be used to identify gaps in developmental sequence in older children and adults, to indicate the need for in-depth assessment or serve as a treatment guide.

POPULATION: Children from birth to 15 months in sections 1 and 2 (prehension patterns), children from 1 to 6 years in section 3 (drawing and writing skills); the 15-month level can be considered a maturity level and therefore an approximate norm for assessing older children. EDPA-S is intended for use with subjects ages 15 months through adulthood. (It has not been field tested.)

SETTING OR POSITION: Subject is supine, prone, or sitting, depending on the test item and according to instructions.

MATERIALS OR TOOLS: Developmental Hand Dysfunction (2nd Edition): Theory, Assessment, and Treatment (manual), assessment protocol and scoring sheets, pencil, graded wooden dowels and cubes, edible pellets, large and small containers, pencil, crayon, yarn and thread, and kit container.

METHOD: The assessment consists of 341 norm components organized into three developmental sequence clusters: involuntary arm–hand patterns (positional/reflexive), voluntary movements (cognitively directed), and prewriting skills, based on the author's theoretical model. (EDPA-S consists of 128 components.) Part One of the test contains the formal test items. For each item, stimulus is presented and/or subject is observed. Right and left hand scores are recorded as normal or well-integrated (+), not present (-), or emerging or abnormal (±). Drawings illustrate each developmental level. Part Two involves translating scores into developmental levels for each cluster. Part Three yields an overview of the child's function in terms of involuntary, voluntary, and prewriting skills.

INTERPRETATION: The interpretation of scores indicates developmental levels, delays, gaps, and intervention needs.

RELIABILITY: Interrater reliability of an earlier version ranged from .71 to .95, based on 16 raters viewing four videotaped evaluation. Intraclass correlations ranged from .41 to .85 (all significant at .001 level). Test–retest reliability studies are needed. EDPA-S has not yet been tested.

VALIDITY: Content validity is based on inclusion of virtually all defined prehension patterns with consideration of the constructs of developmental theory; further construct and discriminant validity studies are needed.

SOURCE: Published by: Therapy Skill Builders, 1994, a division of Psychological Corporation, 555 Academic Court, San Antonio, TX 78204-2498. Tel: 800-228-0752; Fax: 800-232-1223.

SAMPLE: Release of the Dowel or Cube (Supine, Prone, or Sitting)

       L R

4 Months   Mutual fingering in midline, preparation for **transfer**

3 Months   Involuntary release after sustained grasp, with awareness (eyes alert)

COST: $

❑ Erhardt Developmental Vision Assessment (EDVA) and Short Screening Form (EDVA-S)

AUTHOR: Rhoda Priest Erhardt, MS, OTR

FORMAT: Behavior rating scale.

PURPOSE: This test is designed to evaluate visuomotor development and to identify delays, gaps in skill sequences, and inappropriate patterns. Baseline levels may be obtained suggesting specific intervention needs. The screening test is intended to indicate the need for complete diagnostic ophthalmic evaluation.

POPULATION: Normal visual development from birth to 6 months is described; the author recommends the 6-month level as an approximate norm for assessing older children.

SETTING OR POSITION: Room lighting is described for different items as needed; some items require a distance of 6 feet. Testing is done in the subject's most stable position, sitting or semi-reclining; other required positions are described (eg., supine, sidelying)

MATERIALS OR TOOLS: EDVA text (Developmental Visual Dysfunction: Models for Assessment and Management) and pencil; common items are recommended such as light and sound sources and targets for testing.

METHOD: The test consists of 271 items organized into 7 clusters, primarily testing Involuntary Visual Patterns (reflexive) and Voluntary Eye Movements (cognitively directed). The responses are arranged developmentally from fetal to mature (up to 6 months). In each item, a stimulus is presented by an assistant and/or observation made for each eye, and responses are rated according to a scoring key, such as normal well-integrated (+), emerging (±), not present (-). Blinks per minute are recorded. No verbal directions are needed.

EDVA-S is a preliminary version recommended as a quick screening test for ages 6 months through adulthod. It consists of 67 norm components of permanent vision patterns. Scoring is the same as the EDVA.

INTERPRETATION: Developmental level for each cluster is recorded on the scoresheet, yielding a final estimated developmental level in months (fetal through 6). Pattern components indicate gaps in skill sequences, developmentally inappropriate patterns, and needs for intervention. Developmental levels give baseline levels, significant delays, and track progress. Any EDVA-S component scored (-) or (±) indicates the need for full EDVA evaluation.

RELIABILITY: Twenty trained raters scored a video-taped assessment and compared ratings with the test author to determine interrater reliability of the preliminary version; percent of agreement for the entire test averaged 80–90, ranging from 63–86% among clusters. Intraclass correlations averaged .535, with all correlations significant to the .001 level. Test–retest reliability studies are needed.

VALIDITY: Content validity is based on an extensive literature search yielding a comprehensive representation of nearly all visual-motor behaviors organized along a theoretical heierarchy. A concurrent study of reflex and voluntary eye movements in periodic videotapes of five normal infants corroborated the developmental sequences. Further construct and discriminant validity studies are suggested.

SOURCE: Published by: Therapy Skill Builders, 1990, a division of Psychological Corporation, 555 Academic Court, San Antonio, TX 78204-2498. Tel: 800-228-0752; Fax: 800-232-1223.

SAMPLE: GAZE SHIFT (**VISUAL RELEASE**)

6 months **Scans** 3 or more targets within **all focal lengths** quickly and accurately
Eyes move independently from **head** to shift gaze...

COST: $

❏ *FirstSTEP* Screening Test for Evaluating Preschoolers

AUTHOR: Lucy J. Miller, PhD, OTR

FORMAT: Performance-based checklist and rating scales.

PURPOSE: This brief screening test is designed to identify preschool children at risk for developmental delays in the five areas mandated by Individuals with Disabilities Education Act (IDEA). Produced as a companion to the Miller Assessment for Preschoolers (MAP), *FirstSTEP* identifies children in need of more comprehensive evaluation. It is intended for use in individualized large-scale screening.

POPULATION: Children ages 2 years, 9 months through 6 years, 2 months. (Norms are based on 1,443 children at 6-month age intervals and representing a random and stratified sampling of the U.S. population of these ages.)

SETTING OR POSITION: Individual test room is recommended, with minimal distractions, good lighting and ventilation, and enough space for gross motor tasks. For items performed at the table, child and examiner should be seated across from each other in child-size chairs.

MATERIALS OR TOOLS: The kit includes carrying case with manual, Stimulus Booklet, Record Form for each level, Social–Emotional/Adaptive Behavior Booklet, Parent Booklet, and manipulative toys; in addition, a pencil, stopwatch, ruler, coins, and masking tape are needed.

METHOD: *FirstSTEP* consists of 12 subtests divided into three of the five domains: Cognition, Communication, and Motor. Every domain has four subtests or games, each measuring a specific ability (e.g., picture completion, problem solving). The materials, administration, age ranges, and scoring criteria are described in the manual for each item. Items are scored 1 (pass) or 0 (fail); scores are totalled for each domain and converted to composite scores. Administration requires 15 minutes.

The optional Social–Emotional Rating Scale and Adaptive Behavior Checklist contribute important information in the remaining two domains. The Social–Emotional Scale is rated by the examiner based on behavior noted during testing. Adaptive Behavior ratings are based on interviewing the parent or caregiver about daily functioning. The optional Parent/Teacher Scale contributes observations not available during testing. Although these are not part of the Composite Score, raw scores are totalled and recorded for each of the optional scales.

INTERPRETATION: *FirstSTEP* yields three classifications: within acceptable limits, caution (below acceptable limits), and below acceptable limits and needing comprehensive assessment. Cut-off scores are established for each domain and for the composite score, to determine whether performance is in the risk zone. Domain scores further indicate strengths and limitations for treatment planning. The optional scales and check lists may be used to enhance interpretation of the child's performance.

RELIABILITY: Split-half reliability of the domain and composite scores by age group averaged .71–.92. Test–retest reliability over a 1- to 2-week interval for domain and composite scores ranged from .85–.93; classification agreement based on consistency of cut-off scores between the two tests also ranged from .85–.93. Interrater reliability was calculated for classification agreement (.81–1.0) and scaled scores (.77–.96).

VALIDITY: Content validity is based on review by over 50 consultants, evaluations by test examiners during development, and final review by content experts before standardization. Construct validity correlations supported the domains as unique dimensions of ability. Factor analysis confirmed three factors of motor, language, and cognitive ability. Criterion-related studies showed the classification of both normal and delayed children as very accurate for a screening instrument (72%–85%). Concurrent validity studies found positive score correlations between *FirstSTEP* and MAP, WPPSI-R, and with selected scores on Bruininks-Oseretsky, Test of Language Development (TOLD-P:2), Walker Problem Behavior Identification Checklist-R, and Vineland Scales of Adaptive Behavior. Finally, *FirstSTEP* was found to discriminate between normal children and those with cognitive, language, motor, and social–emotional problems.

SOURCES: Published by: The Psychological Corporation, 1993, 555 Academic Court, San Antonio, TX 78204-2498. Tel: 800-228-0752; Fax: 800-232-1223.

Training and instructional videotapes are available from: The Foundation for Knowledge in Development (KID Foundation). Tel: 303-794-1182; Fax: 303-798-2526.

SAMPLE: *Finish Up Game*
Association
Say
Now we're going to play the Finish Up Game. I'm going to tell you something that is not finished. I want you to finish up what I say.
Speaking slowly and clearly, say
A mommy is big; a baby is . . .

COST: $$

❑ Hawaii Early Learning Profile, Revised (HELP®)

AUTHORS: Setsu Furuno, PhD, Katherine A. O' Reilly, PT, MPH, Carol M. Hosaka, MA, Takayo T. Inatsuka, OTR, Toney A. Allman, MA, and Barbara Zeisloft, MS, CCC (instrument); Stephanie Parks, MA (manual)

FORMAT: Nonstandardized scale of developmental skills.

PURPOSE: HELP® is designed as a curriculum-based assessment and intervention program to screen general development in the handicapped infant, using a scale of sequential increments of skills. Multidimensional and family centered, the program attempts to interpret the child's behavior in the context of family and environment.

POPULATION: Children from birth through 3 years who are delayed, have disabilities, or are at risk. HELP® for Preschoolers is available for children ages 3–6 years, with normal or delayed development.

SETTING OR POSITION: Most items are assessed in the child's natural environment during the course of typical daily activities.

MATERIALS OR TOOLS: *Inside HELP®* administration and reference manual, chart, checklist, and activity guide; colored pencils, and many common objects, stimuli or common play equipment are used. A number of other HELP® materials are available, including HELP® for Preschoolers, HELP® Strands, HELP® Family-Centered Interview, HELP® Together software and database, and more.

METHOD: HELP® consists of 685 core developmental skills and behaviors, divided into six areas of function: cognitive, language, gross motor, fine motor, social–emotional, and self-help (regulatory/sensory organization has been added, but is not on the chart). The manual suggests a protocol using an initial warm-up period, structured play, and snack time to complete the assessment. On the HELP® Chart, the evaluator marks each item (+ present, – not present, =/– emerging, and "A" atypical or dysfunctional), as determined by observation or by interview with parent or caretaker. (*Inside HELP®* author explains that the "manual is *not* intended ...to provide standardized evaluation.") Different colored pencils are used for later testing to provide a visual display of the child's functional levels and progress in each developmental area. Explanations of each item are found in the manual; adaptations are suggested for specific disabilities. Assessment may continue over several sessions; only developmentally appropriate items should be administered. For easier recording format, the skills may be transferred from chart to checklist. HELP® Strands is a restructuring of the skills and domains to provide a conceptual framework of 40 developmentally sequenced conceptual strands, which are hierarchical, that is, each skill leads to or builds the foundation for the next one.

INTERPRETATION: Although HELP® is not norm-referenced, HELP® Strands can provide approximate developmental age range levels, document which expected skills are absent, describe the child's behavior, and document dysfunctions. In addition to providing a comprehensive visual profile of a child's function, the HELP® Chart is used with the HELP® Guide and other HELP® materials to plan remedial activities. The manual offers interpretations for cause of difficulty or delay, such as underlying abilities or unrelated interference (e.g., distraction).

REALIABILITY: The 685 skills and behaviors were selected from growth-and-development scales and standardized tests. Although the tool has been field tested extensively in the U.S. and elsewhere, no reliability statistics are offered.

VALIDITY: Face and content validity are demonstrated

by the selection of items by a multidisciplinary team from extensive review of literature and existing scales. Refinement resulted from experience with and critique by experts and users in the U.S. and abroad. No other research or statistics are presented for the instrument or resulting intervention.

SOURCE: Published by: VORT Corporation (1979, 1984, revised 1994), PO Box 60880, Palo Alto, CA 94306. Tel: 415-322-8282; Fax: 415-327-0747.

SAMPLE: Language (18–21 months)

Imitates environmental sounds

Imitates two-word phrases

COST: Manual $; charts ¢; training video $; software and database $$$$.

❒ The INFANIB: A Reliable Method for the Neuromotor Assessment of Infants

AUTHORS: Patricia H. Ellison, MD

FORMAT: Rating scale based on observation and development skills.

PURPOSE: *The Infanib* provides a systematic and reliable neuromotor examination of infants, including primitive reflexes, muscle tone, and posture. It is designed to distinguish normal versus abnormal infants and predict the need for follow-up treatment.

POPULATION: Infants up to 18 months of age, including infants who were premature, exhibit abnormal neuromotor signs, required neonatal intensive care, or have other developmental risk factors.

SETTING OR POSITION: Positions of examiner and infant are described for each item.

MATERIALS OR TOOLS: Manual with scoresheet and pencil, examining table, protractor desireable.

METHOD: *The Infanib* consists of 20 items in five categories: spasticity, head and trunk, vestibular function, legs, French angles. For each item, there is a description and pictures of the test procedure and additional photographs of abnormal and normal test responses. Criteria for scoring on a 3-point scale for each age range are given on the scoresheet. The manual contains discussions of infant neuromotor abnormalities, prognoses over time, other diagnoses, and communication with parents, colleagues, and lawyers. A neurological examination form for newborns and infants and a discharge scoring system are provided for the experienced evaluator to assist in predicting later neurologic abnormality.

INTERPRETATION: The scoresheet yields factor scores and a total score. The degree of normality/abnormality (transient or not) is based on the total score for the subject's correct gestational age. The examiner notes the category of abnormality, such as spastic hemiparesis or hypotonia.

RELIABILITY: Internal consistency is high for the factors and for the total scores at two different ages: .88 for infants $\leq$ 7 months, .93 for infants $\geq$ 8 months, and .91 for all subjects. In a study of 65 infants, each tested twice by two examiners, test–retest and interrater reliability were very high (.95 and .97, respectively).

VALIDITY: Factor analysis was used to group the 20 items into five factors (factor loadings range from .61 to .89). In a study of 243 infants tested at 6 and 12 months, spasticity and the head and trunk subscales at 6 months were highly predictive of cerebral palsy at 12 months (86.8 and 87.1, respectively). According to the author, concurrent validity is based on comparing total scores with impressions of the subjects by experienced examiners; no data are presented on this.

SOURCE: Published by: Therapy Skill Builders, 1994, a division of Psychological Corporation, 555 Academic Court, San Antonio, TX 78204-2498. Tel: 800-228-0752; Fax: 800-232-1223.

SAMPLE: Scarf Sign

> ...The examiner holds the arm near the elbow and moves it across the chest as far as it will move easily, without using force. The angle is measured between an imaginary line dropped from the armpit and the upper arm (with the armpit as the fulcrum). ...

COST: $$

❑ Milani-Comparetti Motor Development Screening Test, Third Edition Revised

AUTHORS: Drs. A. Milani-Comparetti and E.A. Gidoni; modified and revised by the Meyer Children's Rehabilitation Institute

FORMAT: Checklist based on observation of behavior.

PURPOSE: This test is designed to provide a quick and simple method for early identification of neuromotor delays or deficits in children. By examining the integration of primitive reflexes and emergence of volitional movement against gravity, it offers a quantitative and qualitative summary of motor development. It is intended for use in routine health exams and clinics.

POPULATION: Children from birth to 2 years of age. (Standardization sample of revised version consisted of 312 health children, ages 1–16 months, from Omaha area clinics, daycare centers, and homes.)

SETTING OR POSITION: Position described for each item.

MATERIALS OR TOOLS: Scoring chart and manual, pencil, and a firm cushion.

METHOD: The test consists of 27 motor behaviors representing 2 categories: evoked responses (e.g., righting reactions and primitive reflexes) and spontaneous behaviors (e.g., sitting or crawling). Each item has a description of performance expected at different age levels; only age-appropriate items are administered. The examiner positions or manipulates the child as described and scores the observed response by marking along the timeline for each item on the chart. The scoring method compares the child's age with the item age level to determine delays. Additional observations that are significant should be noted off the score form. The test requries 10–15 minutes. Infants suspected of deviation should be retested several times; key ages for examination are offered.

INTERPRETATION: The test yields a graphic profile of the child's motor development for comparison with age norms. Any child with significant delay and/or asymmetry should be further evaluated. The screening tool should be used cautiously for diagnosis or program recommendations. (Additional scoring methods have been developed to distinguish among normal, transiently abnormal, and abnormal infants from 6–16 months; and among delays ranging from 1/2 to > 3 months.)

RELIABILITY: Interrater reliability was based on videotaped administrations scored by 3 therapists and mean precent of agreement ranged from 89–95% (highest in the 9–16 month age range). Test–retest reliability over a 5- to 7-day interval demonstrated mean percent agreement for test items of 82–100%.

VALIDITY: Content validity based on extensive review of literature and clinical observation is apparent from its wide acceptance by physicians and therapists. Further validity studies for the revised version are in progress. The original form was found to accurately identify normal children at 3 months (78%) and 6 months (89%). Preliminary evidence of accurately identifying abnormal infants and of correlating scores with Psychomotor Development Index and Baylet Scles of Infant Development is summarized.

SOURCE: Published by: Meyer Children's Rehabilitation Institute (1977, revised 1992), 600 S. 42nd Street, University of Nebraska Medical Center, Omaha, NE 68131. Tel: 402-559-6467.

SAMPLE: Age in months 1 2 3 4 5 6 7 8 9 10 11 12 13 14
       Body lying supine
       Hand grasp
       Foot grasp

COST: $; training video $$. Formal training is available on request.

❑ Miller Assessment for Preschoolers (MAP)

AUTHOR: Lucy Miller, PhD, OTR

FORMAT: Standardized task performance screening tool; includes nonstandardized supplemental observations form.

PURPOSE: The instrument provides a statistically sound, short, comprehensive screening to determine developmental status and identify moderate (not obvious) delays. Further research may prove it to identify children at risk for school-related difficulties.

POPULATION: Children, aged 2 years, 9 months to 5 years, 8 months; not indicated for severely handicapped children. (Norms are based on a sample of 1,204 children randomly selected according to the 1970–1977 U.S. population census.)

SETTING OR POSITION: Well-lit room at least 2 x 4 yards, with small carpet available.

MATERIALS OR TOOLS: Two or three child-size chairs and table, test kit (includes manual, cue sheets, score sheet, record booklet, scoring transparency and notebook, and test materials), stopwatch.

METHOD: The MAP contains 27 core items that vary according to the age of the subject, plus Supplemental Observations (optional) for the clinically experienced examiner. Items consist of simple sensorimotor tasks, visual–spatial tasks, mental manipulations, cognitive and verbal games, and others. Measures are obtained in the following areas: sensory and motor abilities (foundations index and coordination index), cognitive abilities (verbal index and nonverbal index), and combined abilities (complex tasks index). The test should be administered in 30–40 minutes.

INTERPRETATION: The test yields a final score for comparison with the norms. Percentile equivalents for overall performance and for the five performance indexes are provided. Specific strengths and needs can be determined for treatment planning.

RELIABILITY: Interrater reliability was .978 for total score (index scores ranged from .80 to .99). Test–retest reliability indicated .81 of subjects remained in the same scoring category over a 1- to 4-week interval (.72–.94 range of Index scores). Internal reliability was .79 for this fairly heterogeneous test.

VALIDITY: Content validity is based on analysis of developmental levels of items and on factor analysis. Criterion-related validity is based on correlations of test portions with four other standardized tests. Construct validity is based on scores discriminating children with preacademic problems.

SOURCES: Published by: Psychological Corporation, 1982, 555 Academic Court, San Antonio, Texas 78204-2498. Tel: 800-228-0752; Fax: 800-232-1223.

Miller, L. (1983). MAP: A review. *American Journal of Occupational Therapy, 37*(5), 333–340.

SAMPLE:
1. "Can you make a tall building like mine? Make it as big as you can."
2. "Can you draw a picture of a person?"
3. "Can you roll up into a ball?"

COST: $$$$; Training videotape available.

❏ NCAST (Nursing Child Assessment Satellite Training) Feeding and Teaching Scales

AUTHOR: Dr. Kathryn Barnard and Nursing Child Assessment Project (NCAP)

FORMAT: Observation-based binary (yes/no) scale.

PURPOSE: By studying the caregiving environments of infants and young children, children at risk for later developmental problems can be identified as early as possible. The scales provide a systematic method of evaluating caregiver–child interaction in familiar (Feeding) and unfamiliar (Teaching) routines. The scales may be used for screening, repeated assessment, and treatment planning.

POPULATION: NCAST Feeding Scale is designed for parent or caregiver and child between birth and one year. NCAST Teaching Scale is designed for parent or caregiver and child between birth and 3 years. (NCAST Database consists of large samples collected among various groups—ethnic, mother's age, and education, etc.— to approximate norms).

SETTING OR POSITION: Feeding Scale is given in the natural or routine setting of infant's usual feedings. Teaching Scale permits home or clinic setting, with child awake, caregiver available, environment relatively free of distractions, and child positioned for playing with objects and eye-to-eye contact.

MATERIALS OR TOOLS: Manual, scoresheet, and pencil. Teaching Scale requires a kit containing a variety of toys and common activity supplies (e.g., scissors, crayons), and Child Activity Card for caregiver. Manuals are intended to train administrator with videotapes.

METHOD: The Feeding and Teaching Scales each consist of binary observations (76 and 73 items respectively) organized into six conceptually-based subscales, four describing the caregiver's behavior (sensitivity to cues, response to child's distress, and fostering social–

emotional and cognitive growth) and two of the child's behavior (clarity of cues, responsiveness to caregiver).

The Feeding Scale is rated by a passive observer during a routine feeding; thus it varies in duration with the length of the feeding (20 to 30 minutes usually). The Manual recommends methods or adjustments to maximize the score.

The Teaching Scale requires the caregiver to teach an unfamiliar task to the child, selected from a developmentally graded list of activities.

Both scales utilize a minimum of standard instructions. A scoresheet is completed by checking yes or no for each item and noting ethnic identity of the mother. Yes answers are totalled for each subscale and for Infant Total and Parent/Caregiver Total. The manuals include lengthy scoring guidelines. Training is required by the University of Washington in order to purchase and use the Scales; certification is also available.

INTERPRETATION: Scores based on child's age and caregiver's ethnic identity are significant when they fall below the 10% cutoff level, indicating the need for a repeat or additional assessment.

RELIABILITY: Test–retest reliability is high for Total Parent score (Feeding .75, Teaching .85) and lower for Total Infant Score (Feeding .51, Teaching .55), demonstrating greater stability for parent than infant scores. This may partially reflect infant's developmental change between testings as well as inconsistency in infant's behavior.

VALIDITY: Content validity is demonstrated by items written to reflect concepts of Dr. Barnard. Correlations between NCAST total scores and relevant subscale scores on the HOME Scale, with IQ scores on Bayley Mental Developmental Index, and between Feeding

Scale and other newborn assessment scores demonstrate concurrent validity. Evidence of predictive validity is summarized comparing NCAST scores and later standardized test scores (Bayley, WPPSI, Preschool Language Scale). Extensive studies of discriminant validity are summarized comparing scores of different groups of mothers (e.g., ethnic groups, maternal characteristics such as age and education, presence of substance abuse, etc.) and infants (temperaments, presence of physical or social risk factors, etc.), and interventions and their outcomes.

SOURCE: NCAST Publications (1972, revised 1994), University of Washington, CDMRC, WJ-10, Seattle, WA 98195. Tel: 206-543-8528.

SAMPLE: Sensitivity to Cues   yes/no
    Caregiver varies the intensity of verbal stimulation during feeding.
    Caregiver praises child's successes or partial successes.

COST: $$$ for teaching kit, manuals, and training.

❑ Neonatal Behavioral Assesment Scale (2nd edition) (NBAS)

AUTHORS: T. Berry Brazelton, MD

FORMAT: Behavioral rating scale.

PURPOSE: Designed primarily as a research tool, NBAS was designed to score the baby's interactive behavior and response to the environment. Early behavioral evaluation helps examine the development of the infant–caregiver relationship, cross-cultural differences, and nature vs. nurture contributions to child development.

POPULATION: Newborn infants from 36–44 weeks gestational age; suggestions are made for younger preterm babies and those on supports. (Mean scores are based on expected behavior of full-term normal Caucasian infants, of average weight, in the 3rd day of life.)

SETTING OR POSITION: Quiet, semi-darkened room with a temperature of 72–80° F.

MATERIALS OR TOOLS: Instructions and record forms, and a pencil; in addition, a flashlight, rattle, bell, colored ball, and sterile pin are needed.

METHOD: NBAS consists of 28 behavioral responses and 18 reflex items in 7 clusters: habituation, orientation, motor performance, range of state (of consciousness), regulation of state, autonomic regulation, and reflexes. The exam is administered in an interactive manner, that is, the examiner uses facial expression, gesture, and manual manipulation in response to the infant's behavior in order to elicit the best behavior. Behavioral items are scored according to written criteria on a 9-point scale, and elicited reflex responses on a 0 (not elicited) to 3 (high) scale; either mid-point or 9 on the scales are the norm. Subjects must be between feedings and in the state required for administering each item, beginning with asleep, covered, and dressed and progressing to wide awake; if not possible, items must be omitted and noted. Repeated testing is optimal, but if one test is given, it should be administered after the third day of life. Administration requires 20–30 minutes, with 15 minutes for scoring immediately afterwards. Supplementary items are provided for use with premature infants under 36 weeks of gestational age. Training films and sessions at training centers are needed for reliable testing.

INTERPRETATION: The results give an estimate of how well the newborn is functioning in the adjustment to normal daily stresses. The degree of variability of the infant's state is indicative of the capacity for self-organization. Cluster scores identify which areas of behavior are clinically worrisome.

RELIABILITY: Experience with neonatal assessment and training to elicit optimal response is recommended to achieve interrater reliability level of 90%. Test–retest reliability is questionable as day-to-day stability in a newborn is expected to be low.

VALIDITY: The 7-cluster system noted above is conceptually and empirically based, using factor analysis and other means of organizing the data. Studies comparing newborn scores with later scores (NBAS, Bayley) and with maternal interaction demonstrate NBAS capability to predict behavioral development in the infant as well as early identification of developmental problems. Performance on NBAS has been significantly associated with specific prenatal and labor conditions.

SOURCE: Published by Mac Keith Press, London, 1995. Obtain from U.S. distributor: Cambridge University Press, 40 W. 20th Street, New York, NY 10011. Tel: 800-872-7423.

SAMPLE: Alertness (4 [state] **only**)

1 Inattentive—rarely or never responsive to direct stimulation.
5 When alert, responsiveness of moderate duration—response may be delayed and can be variable.
9 Always alert for most of exam. Intensely and predictably alert.

COST: $ for the book; this does not include training or training tapes.

❑ The Neurological Assessment of the Preterm and Full-term Newborn Infant

AUTHORS: Lilly and Victor Dubowitz

FORMAT: Rating scale based on observation of behavior.

PURPOSE: This instrument was developed to provide a simple, brief neurological examination of newborn infants that can be used in routine assessment. It is intended for sequential evaluation, comparison of preterm with full-term infant behavior, and detection of neurological deviations and their resolution.

POPULATION: Healthy as well as ill preterm and full-term infants within the first few days of life. (Sample consisted of 500 babies tested over 2 years.)

SETTING OR POSITION: Position is described for each item. Setting is assumed to be in nursery or neonatal unit; infant may be in incubator and/or ventilated.

MATERIALS OR TOOLS: Instructions, recording sheets, and a pencil; in addition, optometric torch, "telephone" rattle, and red woolen ball are used.

METHOD: The test consists of 33 items in 4 categories: habituation, movement and tone, reflexes, and neurobehavioral observations. Clear directions for eliciting each item are given on the recording sheet, followed by descriptions of the 5 (or fewer) grades of response, with diagrams when possible. The items are sequenced, beginning with those administered to the infant in a quiet or sleep state, followed by items not influenced by state, and finally those behavioral items

administered to the fully awake infant. The state of the infant is recorded for each item according to Brazelton's 6 gradings of state; comments and asymmetry are also noted. Items are graded on a 5-point scale from minimum to maximum response. The test requires 10–15 minutes.

INTERPRETATION: The assessment yields a pattern of responses to reflect different aspects of neurological function. This pattern is intended as objective documentation of various clinical signs in order to identify deviations for diagnosis.

RELIABILITY: The authors report good reliability between pairs of observers examining the baby independently.

VALIDITY: The assessment was based on extensive review of literature and neonatal examinations. The authors refer to studies comparing full-term infants on days 1 and 5, and full-term with preterm infants of varying gestational ages. The authors describe studies of infants with pathological conditions, the neurological signs exhibited, and the prognosis as documented by serial testing.

SOURCE: Published in: *Clinics in Developmental Medicine,* no. 79, Spastics International Medical Publications, New York, Cambridge University Press, 1981. Obtain from: Cambridge University Press, 40 W. 20th Street, New York, NY 10011. Tel: 800-872-7423.

SAMPLE:

VISUAL ORIENTATION (state 4) To red woollen ball.	Does not focus or follow stimulus.	Sustained fixation; follows vertically, horizontally, and in circle.

COST: $

❏ Newborn Individualized Developmental Care and Assessment Program (NIDCAP)

AUTHOR: Heidelise Als, PhD

FORMAT: Checklist based on observation of behavior.

PURPOSE: Systematic, naturalistic observation of the infant in the nursery or home offers information about the infant's response to environmental input and caregiving routines. This method is appropriate for newborns who are not ready for evaluation by handling, and offers caregiving suggestions and environmental modifications as well as support to the infant's family. (Based on the same research theories as the Assessment of Preterm Infants' Behavior, the NIDCAP is less specialized and more widely available for use.)

POPULATION: Newborns at high risk for developmental compromise. (Sample of 40 low-birthweight infants in a neonatal intensive care unit in Stanford, California who were evaluated and treated with individualized developmentally oriented care.)

SETTING OR POSITION: The nursery (hospital) or home, in the usual setting and position of the infant.

MATERIALS OR TOOLS: Manual, observation package with recording and summary sheets, pencil with eraser, clipboard, and stopwatch.

METHOD: The observation sheets are organized as a frequency checklist in which the infant is observed continuously, and specific behaviors are checked off in 2-minute time intervals. The checklist consists of 91 behaviors that are described and categorized as Autonomic/Visceral, State, Motor, and Attention-related. In addition to behavioral data, parametric autonomic data (heart rate, respiratory rate, and oxygen saturation) are sampled every 2 minutes. The infant is observed in three segments: at least 20 minutes before being handled by a caregiver, during a caregiving intervention (e.g., feeding, bathing, blood test), and at least 20 minutes after

caregiving is terminated. The observations are repeated over time, and background data are collected from the infant's records. The observation is summarized by describing predominant behaviors and their relationship to the autonomic data in the three observation segments.

INTERPRETATION: The resulting picture indicates the infant's relative states of self-regulatory balance versus stress, and the level of support or intrusiveness/manipulation that influences them. From this, strategies and environmental and caregiving modifications are developed to reduce stress and enhance stabilization for the infant.

RELIABILITY: Education and training sessions are conducted at a NIDCAP center or by NIDCAP instructors, after which interobserver reliability (> 85% required) is determined between trainee and instructor ratings of a subject. After completion of the training criteria, the trainee is certified to administer the NIDCAP.

VALIDITY: Outcome studies indicate that infants receiving this developmental approach versus standard care demonstrate improved developmental and neuropsychological measures, shorter hospital stay, and improved behavioral performance at 42 weeks postconception. Long-term studies show evidence of improved neuropsychological function and school achievement to age 8 years.

SOURCES: Materials and training information available through the author at: Neurobehavioral Infant and Child Studies (1981, revised 1984), Children's Hospital, 300 Longwood Avenue, Boston, MA 02115. Tel: 617-355-6179; Fax: 617-355-7230; e-mail: love@al.tch.harvard.edu (contact: Geoffrey Love).

Fleisher, B.E., VandenBerg, K., Constantinou, J., Heller,

C., Benitz, W.E., Johnson, A., Rosenthal, A., Stevenson, D.K. (1995). Individualized developmental care for very-low-birth-weight premature infants. *Clinical Pediatrics, 34*(10): 523–529.

SAMPLE: Time: 0–2   3–4   5–6   7–8   9–10
Attention: Fuss
　　　　　　　Yawn
　　　　　　　Sneeze

COST: $$$$ for training and materials; for reliability session $$$.

❑ Pediatric Evaluation of Disability Inventory (PEDI)

AUTHORS: Stephen M. Haley, PhD, PT, Wendy J. Coster, PhD, OTR/L, Larry H. Ludlow, PhD, Jane T. Haltiwanger, MA, EdM, Peter J. Andrellos, PhD

FORMAT: Standardized behavior checklist and rating scale; may include structured interview.

PURPOSE: The PEDI is a comprehensive clinical assessment of functional capabilities and typical performance in young children with disabilities. It is used to detect functional deficits, monitor progress, or evaluate the outcome of a therapeutic program.

SETTING OR POSITION: Location and time that affords respondent privacy without interruption.

MATERIALS OR TOOLS: Manual, score form, pencil, and software program for data entry, and summary score profiles.

METHOD: The PEDI uses observation, interview, and/ or judgment of professionals familiar with the child to assess three domains: self-care, mobility, and social function. The domains are further broken down into functional subunits that make up each task. The score form contains three sections: Functional skills, Caregiver assistance, and Modifications. Functional skill areas (197 items) are marked 0 (unable) or 1 (capable). The Caregiver Assistance Scale (20 items) is rated from 0 (total assistance) to 5 (independent), and the Modifications Scale (20 items) is rated from E (extensive) to N (no modifications). Scoring criteria are given in the manual. Administration requires 20 to 30 minutes by a familiar therapist or teacher, or 45 to 60 minutes via parent interview and use of the checklist. Training with an experienced user is recommended.

INTERPRETATION: PEDI yields two types of summary scores: normative standard scores indicating the child's relative standing in relation to age expectations, and scaled scores indicating child's performance in relation to ease or difficulty of the item (by Rasch analysis). In addition, totals for frequency of modification levels can be calculated. An optional software program also can calculate a fit score, that is, how consistent the child's performance is with the expected domain profile. PEDI identifies children who show patterns of delay in achieving age-appropriate functional abilities. Normative standard scores help to examine clinical change in relation to expected maturational change.

RELIABILITY: Internal consistency among the six scales ranges from .95 to .99. Interrater reliability of data collected from parent responses on the Caregiver Assistance Scales is .96 to .99 and on Modifications, .79 to 1.00. Comparing two observers with parental and clinical team data, reliability ranges from .84 to 1.00, and .74 to .96 in a rehabilitation day program, except for Social Function (.30), which has since been modified.

VALIDITY: Results of questionnaires sent to 31 content experts to evaluate comprehensiveness and representativeness were incorporated into the final PEDI items. Construct validity is demonstrated by age-related changes in scores. Concurrent validity studies compare Battelle Developmental Inventory Screening Test with PEDI Functional Skills Scales (.70–.81) and with PEDI (.80–.97). Scores differentiated between disabled and nondisabled children. PEDI scores may respond to some clinical changes of subjects.

SOURCE: PEDI Research Group, 1992, Department of Rehabilitation Medicine, New England Medical Center Hospital, #75K/R, 750 Washington Street, Boston, MA 02111-1901. Tel: 617-956-5031.

SAMPLE: Outdoor Locomotion: Methods   0 1
Walks, but holds onto objects, caregiver, or devices for support.
Walks without support.

COST: $$ (software $$)

❏ Quick Neurological Screening Test (QNST)

AUTHORS: Margaret Mutti, MA; Harold M. Sterling, MD; Norma V. Spalding, EdD

FORMAT: Screening test using observation of performance tasks.

PURPOSE: The QNST samples a variety of motor, perceptual, and other functions to determine degree of neurological integration as it relates to learning. It is intended for use by psychologists and school personnel to identify individuals with learning disabilities.

POPULATION: Designed for children as young as 5 years, but it is demonstrated to be effective with adolescents and adults, according to the authors. (Sample consists of over 2,000 subjects from under 6 years to over 17 years of age.)

SETTING OR POSITION: Quiet room at least 10 feet square, with a comfortable writing area.

MATERIALS OR TOOLS: Examination kit (manual, cue cards, recording form, pencil, and ballpoint pen).

METHOD: The QNST consists of 15 observed tasks, requiring approximately 20 minutes to administer. The tasks sample motor development and control, motor planning and sequencing, rhythm, spatial organization, visual and auditory perception, balance and cerebellar-vestibular function, and attention. Subtest scores are tabulated for a single total score.

INTERPRETATION: Scores are categorized as either "high" (likely to have learning problems), "Suspicious" (developmental or neurological symptoms noted), or "normal." The pattern of scores can indicate areas for further assessment.

RELIABILITY: Test–retest reliability was .81 with one examiner over a I-month interval. Scores from tests administered by experts correlated with scores by minimally trained teachers (.69).

VALIDITY: Studies are reported comparing high QNST scores with low schoolwork achievement, behavioral problems, and positive medical–neurologic findings by examination. Also QNST scores correlated positively (.51) with the Bender Visual-Motor Gestalt Test. A study by Ingolia, Cermak, and Nelson (1982) confirms the validity of the test with children exhibiting choreoathetoid movements.

SOURCES: Published by: Academic Therapy Publications, 1978, 20 Commercial Blvd., Novato, CA 94949-6191. Tel: 800-422-7249; Fax: 415-883-3720.

Ingolia, P., Cermak, S.A., & Nelson, D. (1982). The effect of choreoathetoid movements on the Quick Neurological Screening Test. *American Journal of Occupational Therapy, 36*(12), 801–807.

SAMPLE: Hand skill:
> Holds pencil clumsily, tightly
> Prints
> Keeps eyes close to paper
> Exhibits observable tremor

COST: $

❏ Vulpe Assessment Battery—Revised (VAB-R)

AUTHOR: Shirley German Vulpe

FORMAT: Criterion-referenced battery of performance tests, behavioral observations, interview, and record review.

PURPOSE: This comprehensive and systematic developmental assessment is used to gather information about a child's functional abilities for early intervention. It provides a method that can be customized for each child to describe, analyze, and profile the range of developmental skills, behavioral characteristics, and treatment/learning needs of the child.

POPULATION: Children functioning between full-term birth to 6 years of age; originally designed for the child who is mentally retarded but appropriate for any children with atypical developmental patterns related to medical or social conditions.

SETTING OR POSITION: Used in multiple settings where the child spends time (home, hospital, school); equipment and directions are given for each item, but selection, preparation, and presentation are flexible and the examiner may adapt these to the subject.

MATERIALS OR TOOLS: Manual, record sheets, and pencil; common toys and equipment are suggested for each item that the examiner must collect (e.g., blocks, ball, scissors, ice cubes, battery-operated vibrator, tuning fork).

METHOD: VAB-R includes three sections: an Assessment of Basic Senses and Functions in 14 areas (e.g., touch, motor planning, dominance); Assessment of Six Domains of Developmental Behaviors: Gross Motor, Fine Motor, Language, Cognitive Processes, Adaptive Behaviors, and Activities of Daily Living (60 skill sequences in all); and an Assessment of the Environment (7 categories of physical environment and caregiver characteristics and needs). There are a total of 1,300 available developmental tasks; those items within the range of child's current level of development should be assessed. VAB-R can be administered in whole or part, in any setting, by any person familiar with the subject or trained in child development. Adaptations are permitted in directions, equipment, and mode of performance to tailor the assessment to the child. Data can be collected from any pertinent source (family interviews, records, direct observation, testing, etc.) in order to establish the child's typical behaviors.

In Basic Senses and Functions, equipment and directions are given for each category; these items are not scored but are recorded as present/absent, normal/abnormal with comments on the quality of performance. For each skill in the 6 domains, the age level and skill sequence being tested are listed, followed by the suggested materials and method to elicit the performance, the 7-point Vulpe Performance Analysis Scale for scoring each item, and comments on information processing (Information Processing Analysis) and activity analysis (Task/Activity Analysis). For each Environment category, specific questions are listed with a discussion of the importance of that area; comments are recorded from interviews and observation. The assessment can be administered to individuals or groups, and a single child can be tested in two 1-hour sessions.

INTERPRETATION: The Vulpe Performance Analysis Scale provides information on the age ranges of performance in each domain and skill sequence, and an analysis of the amount and kinds of environmental supports required to perform each skill successfully. The Vulpe Performance Analysis System identifies problems in task performance and provides prescriptive information to design early intervention programs, modify tasks to adapt to the child's impairments, begin the teaching process, and monitor the child's response. The results are used to develop an Individualized Education Plan, therapeutic treatment plan, customized developmental curriculum, and Individualized Family Service Plan.

RELIABILITY: Three studies of interrater reliability indicate agreement between raters ranging from .87–.95.

VALIDITY: Concurrent validity between Vulpe Second Edition-Gross Motor Scales and Peabody Developmental Motor Scales-Gross Motor Scales is .99. The authors report improved validity is achieved by the extensive field testing and refining of the descriptions and the flexibility of administration to improve each child's performance. Literature review and agreement of experts yielded the placement of items in domains and age levels, as well as relating them to preschool curricula.

SOURCE: Published by: Slosson Educational Publications, Inc., 1994, PO Box 280, East Aurora, NY 14052. Tel: 800-828-4800; Fax: 800-655-3840.

SAMPLE:	Sense/Function	Equipment & Directions	Comments
	Olfaction (smell).	Any nontoxic material with unpleasant odor (e.g., horseradish). Place on one side of child or on the other. From birth, the infant turns away from unpleasant odors smoothly and efficiently. Lack of success indicates a need for further medical evaluation.	

COST: $$

Motor

Assessments

Bruininks-Oseretsky Test of Motor Proficiency

AUTHOR: Robert Bruininks, PhD

FORMAT: Standardized battery of motor performance tasks (long and short forms contained).

PURPOSE: The tool provides a comprehensive index of motor proficiency as well as separate measures of gross and fine motor skills. The short form is a survey of general motor proficiency. The instrument is designed for use by educators, clinicians (suggests treatment programs), and researchers.

POPULATION: Children 4.5 to 14.5 years; requires minimal verbal comprehension and memory recall from subjects. It may be used for a mildly to moderately retarded population, but is not valid for the severely handicapped. (Norms are based on a stratified sample of 800 children selected from 38 schools according to the 1970 U.S. population census.)

SETTING OR POSITION: Distraction-free area, well-lit and ventilated, and large enough for an 18-yard running course.

MATERIALS OR TOOLS: The manual, record forms, and test materials are contained in the test kit. In addition, two chairs and a table, clipboard, stopwatch, and rug or mat are needed. Subject must wear rubber- or crepe-soled shoes.

METHOD: The test is divided into eight subtests: four gross motor tasks, three fine motor, and one combined. Following a pretest to determine arm and leg preference, the long form (46 items requiring 40–60 minutes) or short form (14 items requiring 15–20 minutes) is administered. Raw scores are expressed in time, duration (e.g., number of push-ups), accuracy, or other methods as described; hand or foot preferences are noted.

INTERPRETATION: The test yields three estimates of motor proficiency: gross motor composite, fine motor composite, and battery composite. Wilson et al. (1995) recommend using subtest rather than composite scores for diagnostic purposes (i.e., to identify children with motor problems) and to suggest treatment goals, and to evaluate change according to raw scores as opposed to normative scores.

RELIABILITY: Test–retest reliability is best with Battery Composite Scores (.89 for grade 2, .86 for grade 6). Interrater reliability was measured on the most subjective subtest (visual-motor control) at .90 and .98 median correlations. Wilson et al. (1995) reviewed reliability studies for the Bruininks and concluded that interrater reliability is too limited to generalize to children with motor problems or to other subtests.

VALIDITY: Construct validity is evident by comparisons of test content with other studies of motor ability, relation of scores with age, homogeneity of test items, and discrimination between normal and disabled subjects.

SOURCES: Published by: American Guidance Service, Inc., Publishers Bldg., Circle Pines, MN 55014. Tel: 800-328-2560; Fax: 612-786-9077. (**1978**)

Wilson, B.N., Polatajko, H.J., Kaplan, B.J., & Faris, P. (1995). Use of the Bruininks-Oseretsky Test of Motor Proficiency in occupational therapy. *American Journal of Occupational Therapy, 49*(1), 8–17.

COST: $$$

SAMPLE: Balance: walking forward, heel-to-toe, on balance beam
Bilateral coordination: jumping up and clapping hands
Strength: standing broad jump

❏ Children's Handwriting Evaluation Scale (CHES) and Children's Handwriting Evaluation Scale for Manuscript Writing (CHES-M)

AUTHORS: Joanne Phelps, Lynn Stempel, and Gail Speck; developed at Texas Scottish Rite Hospital, Dallas, Texas (CHES-M: Phelps and Stempel)

FORMAT: Single-task timed rating scale.

PURPOSE: According to the manual, both instruments are designed as reliable and objective methods for measuring rate and quality of penmanship, cursive (CHES) and manuscript (CHES-M). They identify children who require remediation, indicate which areas need help, and monitor improvement or change.

POPULATION: CHES: children in grades 3 to 8; CHES-M: children in grades 1 to 2. (Sample is based on 1,365 students in regular and resource classrooms in Dallas County.)

SETTING OR POSITION: Children are presumed to be seated at desks. They are asked to clear their desks completely.

MATERIALS OR TOOLS: Manual, #2 pencil, sheet of unlined paper printed with the passage to be copied, and for CHES a second sheet of unlined 8 1/2" x 11" paper.

METHOD: CHES and CHES-M are quick, economical, and easy to administer to individuals or groups. Both tests consist of a printed passage (CHES has 197 letters, CHES-M has 57 letters, including most of the letters of the alphabet), which tells a brief story. The passage is read to the children and they are instructed to copy it with the preferred hand, writing as they usually do and as well as they can. The test is stopped (CHES-M) or the place marked (CHES) after 2 minutes.

INTERPRETATION: The passages are scored according to a rate table for speed and according to loosely defined objective criteria for quality. Quality and rate are evaluated on a 5-point scale from very poor to very good (CHES-M on a 10-point scale). Percentile ranges corresponding to the rankings are provided for each grade. A formula for letter-per-minute rate is given. In addition, CHES contains a key for projective interpretation based on principles of graphoanalysis.

RELIABILITY: Interrater reliability among four raters for CHES and three raters for CHES-M ranged from .85–.95 for grades 1–8.

VALIDITY: Face validity is evident. Preliminary data by Reisman (personal communication, 1995; publication pending) indicated that the mean score (35.2%) of nearly 400 children in standard classrooms fell in the satisfactory to poor range, suggesting caution in interpreting CHES scores.

SOURCE: Available from: CHES, 6831 St. Andrews, Dallas, TX 75205. (**CHES 1984; CHES-M 1987**)

COST: $

SAMPLE: Rating general appearance: Copy should be free of excessive strikeovers or erasures. Letters should not be so small or so large that the passage cannot be easily read... .

❐ Crawford Small Parts Dexterity Test

AUTHORS: John E. and Dorothea M. Crawford

FORMAT: Standardized performance test.

PURPOSE: This test is designed to measure fine eye–hand coordination for vocational testing. Although intended to predict job success in industry, it can also be used to assess manual dexterity among the disabled.

POPULATION: Adolescents and adults (norms available for normal, physically disabled, mentally retarded, learning disabled, and student samples).

SETTING OR POSITION: Well-lighted, distraction-free room; subject seated at a table with materials placed on the table as described in manual.

MATERIALS OR TOOLS: Test kit (board, screws, pins, collars, tweezers, and screwdriver), stopwatch.

METHOD: The test consists of two parts: Part I, Pins and Collars, requires subject to use tweezers to insert pins into holes and collars over them; Part II, Screws, requires subject to screw small screws into the metal plate with screwdriver. Although designed as a work-limit test (subject completes entire task and the time required yields the score; generally about 15 minutes), it may be administered as a time-limit test (record number of pins and collars and screws completed in 3 and 5 minutes, respectively). For group administrations, the time-limit method is used. The test yields separate scores for each part.

INTERPRETATION: The scores are compared to the appropriate norms for interpreting manual skill and dexterity and for predicting success in manual jobs.

RELIABILITY: Split-half test reliability is good for both work-limit and time-limit administrations.

VALIDITY: Test scores correlate well with job ratings; data suggest they are predictive of job success. Correlations with other test results vary.

COST: $$$

SOURCE: Published by: Psychological Corporation, 555 Academic Court, San Antonio, TX 78204-2498. Tel: 800-228-0752; Fax: 800-232-1223. (**1956, manual revised 1981**)

❏ Deuel's Test of Manual Apraxia

AUTHORS: Dorothy F. Edwards, Ruthmary K. Deuel, Carolyn Baum, and John C. Morris

FORMAT: Motor performance rating scale.

PURPOSE: The test is designed to identify the presence, type (ideational, ideomotor, and constructional), and severity of apraxia in individuals with dementia. The studies investigate the relationship of apraxia to loss of functional independence.

POPULATION: Older adults with senile dementia of the Alzheimer's type (SDAT). (Sample consisted of 142 participants with SDAT and 113 healthy participants in the Washington University School Memory and Aging Project.)

SETTING OR POSITION: Subject is seated opposite examiner or at a table, depending on the subtest.

MATERIALS OR TOOLS: Test form, paper and #2 pencil, common objects (cup, ball, match, shoe with laces, envelope, lock and key, and flashlight with batteries), and set of colored alphabet blocks.

METHOD: The test consists of 12 to 14 items in each of four sections: imitation of nonsense gestures, pantomime on command, use of actual objects, and block construction. Each item is timed and scored for accuracy from 0 (immediate accurate response) to 4 (no response after two tries). Prompting is permitted after incorrect responses. The test requires approximately 10 minutes.

INTERPRETATION: The first three sections are the basis for the research described here (Edwards et al., 1991). The total apraxia score (the sum of the three subtests) ranges from 0 to 160, with a cutoff score of 31 indicating the presence of apraxia. In normal health subjects, the mean score was 16.7, with a mean score of 125.4 in severe dementia. Cutoff and mean scores also are tabulated for each subtest.

RELIABILITY: In a study using the first three subtests, interrater reliability was established at .81, internal consistency at .92.

VALIDITY: Scores on the Katz ADL Index exhibited high correlations with the total apraxia score (.65) as well as the three subtest scores (.61, .62, .60), indicating a relationship between apraxia and competence in daily living skills.

SOURCES: Edwards, D.F., Deuel, R.M., Baum, C.M., & Morris, J.C. (1991). A quantitative analysis of apraxia in senile dementia of the Alzheimer's type: Stage-related differences in prevalence and type. *Dementia, 2*, 142–149.

Edwards, D.F., Baum, C.M., & Deuel, R.M. (1991). Constructional apraxia in senile dementia: Contributions to functional loss. *Physical and Occupational Therapy in Ceriatrics, 9*(3,4), 53–68.

For more information, contact: Dorothy F. Edwards, PhD, Washington University, 4567 Scott Avenue, St. Louis, MO 63105. Tel: 314-286-1600.

COST: ¢

SAMPLE: Gesture with hands— Seconds Score "Pretend this is a birthday cake. _____ 0 1 2 3 4 I want you to blow the candles out."

❒ Evaluation Tool of Children's Handwriting (ETCH) (Manuscript: ETCH-M and Cursive: ETCH-C)

AUTHOR: Susan J. Amundson, MS, OTR/L

FORMAT: Criterion-referenced single-task timed performance test.

PURPOSE: ETCH is designed to evaluate a child's legibility and speed of writing in various manuscript and cursive writing tasks that simulate those required of a student in school. It can be used in schools, educational centers, pediatric clinics, or hospitals to assist in planning intervention and IEP goal and objectives.

POPULATION: Children in grades 1–3 (ETCH-M) and 3–6 (ETCH-C). (Legible and illegible handwriting samples were taken from 161 children from different states.)

SETTING OR POSITION: Individual administration requires a quiet corner of the classroom or isolated testing room.

MATERIALS OR TOOLS: Test kit includes Wall Charts for far-point copying, Task Sheets for near-point copying, Peephole Score Card, Quick Reference sheets, response booklets, score sheets, and manual; and a pencil.

METHOD: ETCH examines speed and legibility of manuscript and the more complex cursive writing. Tasks include writing alphabet and numerals from memory, near- and far-point copying, manuscript-to-cursive transition, dictation, and sentence composition. Speed is measured in letters per minute, and legibility is measured in percentages of numeral, letter, and word legibility. Legibility components (letter formation, spacing, size, alignment) as well as sensorimotor skills related to the handling of the paper and writing tool are examined. Classroom observations include psychosocial skills, attention, and school behavior. Administration requires 15–25 minutes, with 10–20 minutes for scoring.

INTERPRETATION: Each task is scored individually acccording to objective criteria and compiled for a total score, providing a quantitative and qualitative basis for educational and intervention planning. Legibility and speed performance, the foundations of functional written expression, are used to obtain baseline data and to monitor progress.

RELIABILITY: Interrater reliability between raters experienced and inexperienced with ETCH-M are given: total letters (.90), total numbers (.87), and total words (.75). Scoring competency is achieved by the examiner through tutorials and competency quizzes in the manual. ETCH-M test–retest studies are in progress.

VALIDITY: Approximately 30 practitioners contributed to development and pilot testing over 5 years. Literature and current assessments are extensively reviewed.

SOURCE: Published by: O.T. KIDS, 53805 East End Road, Homer, AK 99603. Tel: 907-235-0688; Fax: 907-235-7564. (**1995**)

COST: $$

SAMPLE: NEAR-POINT COPYING—MANUSCRIPT
Task
This task will require the child to write a five-word sentence in manuscript from a nearby manuscript model. The model sentence is, "Ships flew by the moon."

❐ Functional Test for the Hemiparetic Upper Extremity

AUTHORS: Dorothy J. Wilson, OTR, FAOTA, Lucinda L. Baker, MS, PT, and Judith A. Craddock, OTR

FORMAT: Battery of performance tasks.

PURPOSE: The test is designed to evaluate, in an objective fashion, the integrated function of the total hemiparetic upper extremity of the adult. It is intended for use as a clinical tool in initial evaluation and for measuring progress.

POPULATION: Hemiparetic adults. (Sample consisted of 52 hemiparetic adult patients admitted to the stroke service of a large rehabilitation hospital).

SETTING OR POSITION: Varies with item, although designed for use in a variety of settings (bedside, clinic).

MATERIALS OR TOOLS: Protocol booklet, scoresheet, and pencil; detailed description of common materials required accompanies test instructions.

METHOD: The test consists of 17 motor activities graded by degree of difficulty into 7 levels (level 7 is the most complex). Each item is graded on a pass/fail basis, most within a given time limit. Each task has standardized procedures, including equipment and position of subject, and grading criteria. Administration requires 30 minutes or more.

INTERPRETATION: The test yields a single score, indicating level of function achieved.

RELIABILITY: Interrater reliability is .976, raters grading all scores within one item of each other.

VALIDITY: Although there are no comparable tests available, concurrent validity is supported by correlations with several objective upper extremity measures.

SOURCES: Available from: Los Amigos Research and Education Institute, Inc., PO Box 3500, Downey, CA 90242. Tel: 310-940-7165; Fax: 310-803-5569. (**1984**)

Wilson, D. J., Baker, L.L., & Craddock, J.A. (1984). Functional Test for the Hemiparetic Upper Extremity. *American Journal of Occupational Therapy, 38*(3), 159–164.

COST: ¢

SAMPLE: Level 4: Stabilize a jar
Stabilize a package
Wringing a rag

❑ Hand-Tool Dexterity Test

AUTHORS: Publisher acknowledges research contributions of multiple authors

FORMAT: Standardized performance task.

PURPOSE: The test is designed as a measure of proficiency in using ordinary mechanics' tools. This proficiency is described as a combination of aptitude and achievement based on past experience in handling tools. The test attempts to isolate manipulative skill independent of intellectual abilities.

POPULATION: Adolescents (high school students) and adults. (Norms are presented for industrial applicants and employees, adults in vocational training programs, handicapped adults in vocational evaluation and rehabilitation programs, and mentally retarded adults and students.)

SETTING OR POSITION: Test frame is mounted securely on a sturdy table or workbench 34 inches above the floor, allowing a 36" by 24" workspace, with nuts, bolts, and tools placed by the frame as designated.

MATERIALS OR TOOLS: Test frame with three sizes of nuts and bolts; two adjustable wrenches; stopwatch.

METHOD: The test consists of one assembly task: removing nuts and bolts from one side of the test frame with the appropriate tools , and remounting them on the other side of the test frame. It is a speed test: The score is the amount of time it takes from picking up the wrench until the last bolt is tightened.

INTERPRETATION: Raw scores are converted to percentile scores. Normative tables are offered for comparison with numerous categories of students and workers, some broken down by gender or by Caucasian versus minority affiliation.

RELIABILITY: Test–retest reliability with one-to-five-day intervals was .81 in a study of 153 high school dropouts, and .88 in a second study of 75 vocational high school students with immediate retest.

VALIDITY: In two studies of experienced mechanics and trainees in technical programs, test scores were compared to supervisors' ratings and ranged from .07 to .19 in the first and -.45 on the second. Earlier studies comparing test scores with job ratings or school grades yielded correlations ranging from .14 to .51. In comparisons of Hand-Tool test scores with other test scores, higher correlations were found with other measures of dexterity, with a total range of (-.23) to .79.

SOURCE: Available from: Lafayette Instrument, 3700 Sagamore Parkway North, PO Box 5729, Lafayette, IN 47903. Tel: 800-428-7545; Fax: 317-423-9077. (**Revised from 1965**)

COST: $$

SAMPLE: The idea of this test is to remove all these bolts from this upright and place them on corresponding rows on the other upright...It is quicker to loosen all the nuts on each row before putting down your tools...

❏ Jebsen Hand Function Test

AUTHORS: Robert H. Jebsen, MD, Neal Taylor, MD, Roberta B. Trieschmann, PhD, Martha J. Trotter, BA, and Linda A. Howard, BA

FORMAT: Standardized norm-based performance test.

PURPOSE: This simple test was designed to assess the effective use of the hands in everyday activity by performing tasks representative of functional manual activities. It provides objective measures for comparison with norms to assess capabilities and the effectiveness of treatment.

POPULATION: Children and adults, over 5 years of age. (Adult sample consisted of 360 normal subjects, ages 20–94, and 26 patients with stable hand disorders; children's sample consisted of 66 normal children, ages 6–19 years, and 20 children with stable hand disabilities.)

SETTING OR POSITION: Subject is seated at a table in a well-lighted room.

MATERIALS OR TOOLS: Table and chair, pencil, stopwatch, and a collection of common objects (paper, pencil, clipboard, index cards, coffee can, pennies, paper clips, bottle caps, kidney beans, spoon, wooden board, C-clamp, wooden checkers, tape). A kit is available that includes all materials and instructions in a carrying bag.

METHOD: The test consists of 7 simple manual tasks designed to sample or simulate functional hand tasks. They are: writing a short sentence (eliminated for 6- to 7-year-olds), card turning (simulated page turning), picking up small common objects, simulated feeding, stacking checkers, and picking up light and heavy large objects. For each item, a brief description and standardized instructions are given, with the nondominant hand tested before the dominant hand. All items are timed, most requiring about 10 seconds per item by normal adults.

INTERPRETATION: Item scores (and total scores for children) are compared to the normative tables according to age and sex. Reassessments allow the subject to be compared to own scores as well as to the norms in order to measure the effectiveness of intervention.

RELIABILITY: Because the range of scores is so restricted in the normal population, test–retest reliability was examined for the patient groups only, demonstrating the absence of a practice effect (subtest correlations ranged from .60–.99 for disabled adults and .87–.99 for disabled children, with total score correlations of .98–.99 for the children).

VALIDITY: The discriminative ability of the test to determine various degrees of hand function within the disabled sample showed a wide range of mean scores among the patient sample, indicating a range of functional ability. Content validity is questioned by Mathiowetz (1993) who suggests that the subtests are poor simulations of the actual tasks, but whether they are representative of manual ability in general is not addressed.

SOURCES: Kit may be purchased from: Sammons Preston Inc., PO Box 50710, Bolingbrook, IL 60440-5071. Tel: 800-323-5547; Fax: 800-547-4333.

Jebsen, R.H., Taylor, N., Trieschmann, R.B., Trotter, M.J., & Howard, L.A. (1969). An objective and standardized test of hand function. *Archives of Physical Medicine & Rehabilitation*, (June), 311–319.

Mathiowetz, V. (1993.) Role of physical performance component evaluations in occupational therapy functional assessment. *American Journal of Occupational Therapy*, 47, 228.

Taylor, N., Sand, P.L., & Jebsen, R H. (1973). Evaluation of hand function in children. *Archives of Physical Medicine & Rehabilitation*, 54, 129–135.

COST: ¢ (requiring collection of own materials); kit $$$

SAMPLE: SIMULATED FEEDING

Instructions—"Take the teaspoon in your left hand please. When I say 'Go,' use your left hand to pick up these beans one at a time with the teaspoon and place them in the can as fast as you can... ."

❏ Minnesota Handwriting Test (MHT)

AUTHOR: Judith Reisman, PhD, OTR

FORMAT: Single-task timed performance test.

PURPOSE: The MHT was developed to quantify selected aspects of students' printed handwriting samples in order to support other subjective judgments of poor quality and slow rate. It can help identify students with poor manuscript printing and document progress after intervention.

POPULATION: First and second grade students. (Norms are based on a sample of 1,100 first and 926 second graders from 9 states.)

SETTING OR POSITION: Not prescribed; it is assumed that the subject is sitting at a child-size desk or table.

MATERIALS OR TOOLS: Manual with instructions and training exercises for scoring in both D'Nealian and standard manuscript styles, clear plastic ruler with 1/16- and 1/8- inch measurements, timer, and pencil with eraser. (Test forms in both styles may be photocopied.)

METHOD: MHT is a near point copy test in which words are copied from a preprinted sample onto marked lines below the sample. The words are presented in mixed order to eliminate the effect of reading ability on speed and memory. The test is timed for 2.5 minutes for the speed score (i.e., number of letters copied), then time is allotted to complete the sample. Quality is measured in five categories: legibility, form, alignment, size, and letter/word spacing; each letter is scored up to 5 points, one for each category. Students may be tested individually or in groups; standard verbal directions are given, and nonverbal cues may be used during individual testing.

INTERPRETATION: In the preliminary version of the MHT, the raw scores are compared to the mean and standard deviations of the normative tables according to age, grade, and school quarter, as well as gender, handedness, and type of print. The author suggests that observation of posture, pencil grip, attention to task, and comparison to typical school work support the evaluation.

RELIABILITY: Interrater reliability between experienced scorers was .99 for the total sample, with a range of .90 on form (more subjective judgment) to .99 for alignment and size (ruler measurements). Interrater reliability between inexperienced raters was .98, with a range of .87 to .98. Intrarater reliability (scoring same tests twice) was .96–.98. Test–retest reliability over a 1-week interval was .72 for accuracy (ranging .58–.94), and .50 for speed (ranging .47–.67), indicating an influence of other variables.

VALIDITY: Content validity is based on literature review and consultation with primary grade teachers to arrive at scoring categories. In concurrent validity studies of first and second graders in regular and special education classes, MHT scores correlated with Visual-Motor Integration Test (.32), Children's Handwriting Evaluation Scale-Manuscript (.43), and Test of Visual-Motor Skills (.37 for 2nd graders, .62 for 1st graders, .76 for special education students not referred to occupational therapy [OT], and .89 for special education students receiving OT). Only the latter supports discriminant validity in that children requiring therapy demonstrate poor handwriting scores on the MHT.

SOURCE: Publication pending. Contact author for information: Judith Reisman, PhD, OTR Box 388 UMHC, Minneapolis, MN 55455. E-mail: reism001@maroon.tc.umn.edu.; Fax: 612-625-7192.

COST: Undetermined

**SAMPLE: the brown jumped lazy
 fox quick dogs over**

☐ Minnesota Rate of Manipulation Tests (MRMT) and Minnesota Manual Dexterity Test (MMDT)

AUTHOR: None specified (prototype developed in 1933 by University of Minnesota Employment Stabilization Research Institute)

FORMAT: Standardized speed tests.

PURPOSE: The tests are designed to measure manual dexterity, or the speed of gross arm and hand movements during rapid eye–hand coordination tasks. They are used in vocational evaluation to predict performance in general semi-skilled operations. The two versions described appear to be slightly different refinements of the same original instrument.

POPULATION: The MRMT presents norms based on a 1946 sample of 3,000 adults and a second set of tables (1957) based on 11,000 new subjects, generally younger people earlier in their careers. The MMDT states that standard adult norms are applicable to anyone aged 13–15 years and up who can understand the directions.

SETTING OR POSITION: The MRMT specifies that the subject stand at a testing table between 28 and 32 inches in height, the test board 10 inches from the subject's edge of table. (The MMDT does not describe precise positions).

MATERIALS OR TOOLS: Test table, timing device, test board, and blocks (MRMT contains 60 blocks and holes; MMDT contains 58); instructions, recording sheet, and a pencil.

METHOD: Both versions consist of two widely used tests: the Placing Test (blocks placed into holes) and the Turning Test (blocks turned over). The MRMT has three additional tests: the Displacing Test (move blocks to next hole), One-Hand Turning and Placing Test, and Two-Handed Turning and Placing Test. Following practice trials, the subject is scored by totaling the number of seconds it takes to complete each of four trials on each test. (The MRMT allows two, three, or four test trials.) The test may be administered individually or by groups; the latter is preferable as it enhances motivation through competition. Separate procedures are provided for administering the MRMT Displacing Test and Turning Test to the blind.

INTERPRETATION: Raw scores are converted into Composite (MRMT) or Percentile (MMDT) scores. Each version has its own norm charts. A general interpretation of speed percentages is offered for MMDT.

RELIABILITY: Time score correlations are reported for the four tests of the MRMT (ranging from .87 to .95 for two trials and .93 to .97 for four trials), and for the two subtests of the MMDT (.57 between speed of hand and speed of finger movements).

VALIDITY: The MRMT contains data comparing scores with independent supervisor's ratings of workers (ranging from .39 to .67 for four tests) and also between MRMT and Pennsylvania Bi-Manual Work Sample (.46 Placing, .40 Turning). No validity data are reported for the MMDT.

SOURCE: MRMT is published by: American Guidance Service, Inc., Publishers' Building, Circle Pines, MN 55014. Tel: 800-328-2560; Fax: 612-786-9077. MMDT is published by: Lafayette Instrument Co., 3700 Sagamore Parkway North, PO Box 5729, Lafayette, IN 47903. 800-428-7545; Fax: 317-423-4111. (**1969**)

COST: MRMT—$$$; MMDT—$$.

❑ Motor Assessment Scale (MAS)

AUTHORS: Janet H. Carr and Roberta B. Shepherd

FORMAT: Standardized performance scale.

PURPOSE: The MAS was designed to quantitatively measure the motor recovery of stroke patients by using functional tasks. It is a brief and easy instrument to administer, and is used clinically for monitoring progress and for research.

POPULATION: Stroke patients. (Research samples consisted of adult patients with cerebrovascular accidents [CVAs] at various stages of recovery.)

SETTING OR POSITION: Quiet, private room or curtained-off area, administered when patient is alert and dressed.

MATERIALS OR TOOLS: Low wide plinth, stopwatch, polystyrene cup, jellybeans, teacups, rubber ball, stool, comb, pen with top, table, dessert spoon and water, paper, and cylinder.

METHOD: MAS consists of 1 item measuring general muscle tone and 8 motor function items: supine to side lying, supine to sitting at side of bed, balanced sitting, sitting to standing, walking, upper arm function, hand movements, and advanced hand activities. Items are graded according to criteria on a 7-point scale from 0 to 6 (optimal). Subjective information is recorded as comments. Items can be administered in any order, and require approximately 15 minutes or more.

INTERPRETATION: Scores are recorded on a graph, yielding a visual profile of motor function/recovery and tone, and offering immediate feedback to the subject. Items can be readily compared with each other to identify weak areas of function, and progress is easily compared to earlier results.

RELIABILITY: Reliability was determined from video-taped assessments (excluding tone). Test–retest reliability by a single rater with a 4-week interval ranged .87–1.00, with an average correlation of .98. Interrater reliability for the videotaped sessions ranged .89–.99 correlation among raters, with average percent agreement of 87. Interrater reliability for direct observation of patient performance was investigated separately, with total score correlation of .99, items ranging .92–1.00, except for tone (.29), which could not be reliably observed.

VALIDITY: Concurrent validity was demonstrated by total score correlation of .88 with the Fugl-Meyer Assessment, items ranging from .64-.92, except for sitting balance (.28). Poole and Whitney (1988) suggest further studies of the scoring heierarchy.

SOURCES: Published in: Carr, J.H., Shepherd, R.B., Nordholm, L., & Lynne, D. Investigation of a new Motor Assessment Scale for stroke patients. *Physical Therapy,* *65,* 175–180. (**1985**)

Poole, J.L., & Whitney, S.L. (1988). Motor Assessment Scale for stroke patients: Concurrent validity and interrater reliability. *Archives of Physical Medicine and Rehabilitation, 69,* 195–197.

COST: ¢

SAMPLE: Upper-Arm Function

1. Lying, protract shoulder girdle with arm in elevation. (Therapist places arm in position and supports it with elbow in extension.) ... to ...

6. Standing, hand against wall. Maintain arm position while turning body toward wall. (Have arm abducted to 90° with palm flat against the wall.)

❐ Peabody Developmental Motor Scales (PDMS)

AUTHORS: Rhona Folio, EdD and Rebecca Fewell, PhD

FORMAT: Standardized rating scales, based on task performance and observation.

PURPOSE: The test is designed as a comprehensive evaluation of gross and fine motor development in children to determine the level of skill development, identify skills not developed, and plan remediation. In addition, the scales accommodate the special requirements of the severely handicapped population. The instrument was developed by educators for general programming and physical education.

POPULATION: Children, ages 0 to 83 months. (Norms are based on stratified quota sampling of over 1,200 children to represent U.S. population). The test is appropriate for severely and profoundly handicapped children, including those who are deaf-blind.

SETTING OR POSITION: Distraction-free, well-lighted area, with table and chairs, stairs nearby; subject's position for each item is described in manual.

MATERIALS OR TOOLS: Test kit includes manual, activity cards, and fine motor manipulatives; also needed are additional materials specified in manual (balance beam, chair, stairs, and common children's toys).

METHOD: The test consists of 170 items in the Gross Motor Scales and 112 items in the Fine Motor Scales; divided into 17 and 16 age levels, respectively. Testing is begun one level below the child's expected motor age (basal age level) and continues until the child can complete no more than one item in a level (ceiling age level). Each item is scored 0, 1, or 2, according to defined criteria. Administration of the test requires 45 to 60 minutes, or longer with a handicapped child. Instructions are given for group administration.

INTERPRETATION: Cumulative scores can be converted to percentile rank, standard scores, and age-equivalent scores. The test yields a motor development profile. The kit includes a set of activity cards, providing instructional strategies for each test item.

RELIABILITY: Test–retest reliability for the normative sample is good (.95 for Gross Motor, .80 for Fine Motor scales), as is interrater reliability (.97 for Gross Motor, .94 for Fine Motor scales).

VALIDITY: Content validity is based on Harrow's Taxonomy of the Psychomotor Domain (1972). Construct validity is determined by differentiation of scores among chronological ages and between normal children and those with clinical problems.

SOURCE: Published by: The Riverside Publishing Co., 8420 Bryn Mawr Avenue, Chicago, IL 60631-9979. Tel: 800-767-8378. (**1983**)

COST: $$$

SAMPLE:

Level	Item	Child's Position	Directions and Criterion
4–5 months	Holding rattle	Back	Place rattle in child's hand. Say "Shake your rattle." Citerion: Holds and moves rattle for 1 minute.

❐ Purdue Pegboard

AUTHOR: Joseph Tiffin, PhD

FORMAT: Standardized performance tasks.

PURPOSE: This test is designed as a simple and easily administered measure of dexterity in fingertip activity, as well as finger/hand/arm activity. It is intended for use in selecting employees for industrial jobs but has broad clinical application as well.

POPULATION: Adults (standardized on several thousand industrial employees; data accumulated from employers and organized in tables, according to type of work). Normative data have also been collected on children and adolescents, ages 5 to 19 years, in various studies summarized by Mathiowetz, et al. (1986).

SETTING OR POSITION: Seated comfortably at a table, approximately 30 inches high, with pegboard directly in front of test subject.

MATERIALS OR TOOLS: Pegboard equipped with pins, collars, and washers; manual; and stopwatch.

METHOD: The test can be administered individually or in groups, in one trial or three trials. Five scores can be obtained: Right Hand, Left Hand, Both Hands, Right plus Left plus Both Hands, and Assembly. Each task consists of placing pins, collars, and/or washers on pegboard in a 30- or 60-second period.

INTERPRETATION: Score consists of the number of pins or assemblies completed within time limits, which is then compared to the appropriate normative tables.

RELIABILITY: Test–retest reliabilities are reported adequate for one-trial administrations (.60 to .76) but are higher for three-trial administrations (.82 to .91). Later studies confirm this.

VALIDITY: Various studies of predictive validity are summarized, comparing employee scores with production or performance ratings. It is recommended that local studies be carried out for the individual uses of the test.

SOURCES: Available from: Lafayette Instrument Company, 3700 Sagamore Parkway North, PO Box 5729, Lafayette, IN 47903. Tel: 800-428-7545; Fax: 317-423-4111. (**1948, revised 1960**)

Mathiowetz, V., Rogers, S. L., Dowe-Keval, M., Donahoe, L., & Rennells, C. (1986). The Purdue Pegboard: Norms for 14- to 19-year-olds. *American Journal of Occupational Therapy, 40*(3), 174–179.

COST: $$

SAMPLE: Pick up one pin at a time with your right hand, from the right-hand cup. Starting with the top hole, place each pin in the right-hand row.

❑ Roeder Manipulative Aptitude Test

AUTHOR: Wesley S. Roeder

FORMAT: Standardized performance task.

PURPOSE: The Manipulative Aptitude Test is designed to evaluate speed and accuracy of eye, hand, and finger movements. It is used to test the suitability of individuals for employment and upgrading in jobs in which dexterity is a primary requirement. It may be used as part of a vocational test battery for assessment of groups as well as individuals.

POPULATION: Adolescents and adults. (Norms are based on over 4,600 high school students and members of industrial groups in 27 states in the U.S.)

SETTING OR POSITION: Subject is seated comfortably at a table or desk with formboard in a specified position.

MATERIALS OR TOOLS: Styrene-plexiglass performance board with rows of sockets into which nuts are installed, and including receptacles for rods, washers, nuts, caps; in addition, a T-shaped bar is attached to the board for stringing small parts onto it; and a stopwatch.

METHOD: The test consists of four separate timed operations: rod and cap assembly into the board sockets (with dominant hand), and three washer-nut assemblies onto the T-bar (two hands, right hand, left hand). Standardized instructions and time limits (3 minutes or 10 seconds) are provided for each operation. Each assembly is scored by counting the number of pieces (e.g., number of nuts and washers) that are completed for each operation. Raw scores are converted into percentiles and graphed on the profile sheet. Separate instructions are available for individuals versus group administration and for children and others with special needs (e.g., slow learners, handicapped, remedial students).

INTERPRETATION: A Total Manipulative Aptitude percentile may be calculated, with left and right hand dexterity scores. Percentile norms are provided to compare the Total Manipulative Aptitude, right hand, and left hand scores with the normative sample.

RELIABILITY: Test–retest reliability is reported to be .92.

VALIDITY: In studies of electronics assembly workers, correlations between test scores and supervisors' ratings were .42 and .49.

SOURCE: Available from: Lafayette Instrument Co., 3700 Sagamore Parkway North, PO Box 5729, Lafayette, IN 47903. Tel: 800-428-7545; Fax: 317-423-4111. (**1967**)

COST: $$$

SAMPLE: ...PICK UP A ROD IN THIS MANNER (demonstrate) AND, WITH A QUICK TWIST, SCREW IT INTO THE SOCKET AT THE FAR LEFT IN THE TOP ROW. THEN TAKE A CAP (demonstrate) AND, WITH A QUICK TWIST, SCREW THE CAP ONTO THE ROD. ...

❑ Sensorimotor Performance Analysis (SPA)

AUTHORS: Eileen W. Richter, MPH, OTR, FAOTA, and Patricia C. Montgomery, PhD, PT

FORMAT: Criterion-referenced rating scale based on observation of performance.

PURPOSE: SPA is designed to provide a qualitative record of individual performance on gross and fine motor tasks. It is used to analyze underlying sensorimotor components of performance for treatment planning, and to document changes in status.

POPULATION: Ambulatory/mobile developmentally disabled children and adults from age 5 to 21 years; appropriate with severely cognitively impaired or for preschool children with some fine motor tasks eliminated. (Pilot study included 10 normal and 10 trainable mentally retarded children.)

SETTING OR POSITION: Areas of carpeting and of vinyl flooring are needed. Position is prescribed for each item.

MATERIALS OR TOOLS: SPA book and test form, scoring rule, pencil, and materials or equipment generally available in therapy settings (tape, tiltboard, tetherball, pencils, paper, table and chairs, scissors, pellets, bottle, and drawing of "+" and "0").

METHOD: SPA consists of four gross motor and three fine motor tasks broken down into performance components. Therapist instructs subject verbally or by demonstration or prompting to perform task in any manner subject is able. Therapist observes the task and rates each component on a continuum from 0 (unable) to 5 (optimal), representing quality of performance. Items are criterion referenced, scores assigned according to specific criteria of performance. A short Reflex-Testing Assessment is offered for comparison with SPA results. Administration and scoring requires 30 to 45 minutes or less. Administrators should have extensive knowledge of sensorimotor theories and clinical experience in pediatrics.

INTERPRETATION: Scores are transferred to the Scoring Profile to provide a quantitative overview of results that suggests patterns of performance and/or dysfunction. Performance items are grouped according to related sensorimotor components in order to identify areas for intervention. Scores are totalled for each sensorimotor component, with interpretations offered through case examples. "Quick Screening" observations provide subjective comments to support or supplement data.

RELIABILITY: Test–retest reliability on 10 children with a 1-week interval ranged from .89 to .97. Interrater reliability is .76 if categories of asymmetrical tonic neck, symmetrical tonic neck, and tactile processing are eliminated; there is poor agreement in these areas.

VALIDITY: None is demonstrated, except face validity is evident in anecdotal findings that poor SPA performance is indicative of dysfunction. The lack of similar measures precludes concurrent studies according to the authors.

SOURCE: Published by: PDP Products, 12015 N. July Avenue, Hugo, MN 55038. Tel: 612-439-8865. (**1989**)

COST: $

SAMPLE: Kneeling Balance
1. Assumes kneeling
2. Maintains kneeling position
3. Hip stability

❑ Test of Gross Motor Development (TGMD)

AUTHOR: Dale A. Ulrich

FORMAT: Norm- and criterion-referenced performance test.

PURPOSE: The TGMD assesses two specific types of common motor skill process or pattern: locomotor and object control. It is used to identify children with significant problems of gross motor skill development, recommend intervention, measure progress, evaluate intervention programs, and for research involving gross motor development.

POPULATION: Children, ages 3–10 years. (Sample consisted of 909 children in 8 states, representative of the 1980 U.S. Census.)

SETTING OR POSITION: Test environment with minimal distraction, set-up described for each item. Subject should wear rubber soled shoes.

MATERIALS OR TOOLS: Test manual, Student Record Book, masking tape, chalk, or other marking devices, plastic bat, several balls of specified sizes, and a pencil.

METHOD: TGMD consists of 7 locomotor skills and 5 object control skills. Each skill includes 3–4 performance criteria representing a mature pattern of the skill. Following a demonstration and practice trial, the student performs the skill 3 times, and is marked 1 or 0 for each criterion or skill component (1 = successful performance 2 out of 3 times). These scores are added up for locomotor and object control raw subtest scores, then converted to subtest standard scores, percentiles, and a composite quotient representing total gross motor development performance. Comments on behavior or performance during testing are recorded. Testing can be done individually or in groups of two or three children and requires approximately 15 minutes.

INTERPRETATION: Raw scores specify the number of motor behaviors that have been mastered. Tables indicating ages at which skills and components are mastered may assist with recommending specific skill instruction. Percentile rank compares the subject to the age norms, while standard scores allow comparison with other standardized test results. Standard scores are rated from Very Superior to Very Poor for the two skill areas, as well as for the more reliable overall Gross Motor Development Quotient (GMDQ). (Eligibility criteria by scores are given for specialized services through school districts or agencies.)

RELIABILITY: Test–retest reliability on 10 subjects videotaped for scoring by 20 raters achieved generalizability coefficients (see manual) of .95–.99 in all but running (.84), with subtest means of .96–.97. Interrater generalizability coefficients ranged from .77–.99, with means of .95–.97 for 20 raters, .94–.96 for 10 raters, and .86–.87 for 2 raters. For use as a criterion-referenced test in decisions of mastery versus nonmastery of skills, GMDQ cut-off scores were found to be reliable determinations for handicapped and nonhandicapped children.

VALIDITY: The behaviors selected to represent each motor skill were based on motor development literature, review by three content experts, and item analysis to determine the ability of the items to discriminate among high and low scorers. Factor analysis was used to determine that the skills are highly related, supporting the construct of gross motor development. In addition, gross motor skills improved with age (scores correlated with chronological age), and nonhandicapped children exhibited more mature gross motor patterns than mentally retarded children. Finally, test results of children with formal gross motor instruction improved significantly over those of children engaged in free play.

SOURCE: Available from: Pro-Ed, 8700 Shoal Creek Boulevard, Austin, TX 78757-6897. Tel: 512-451-3246; Fax: 800-FXPROED. (1985)

COST: $$

SAMPLE:	Skill	Equipment	Directions	Performance Criteria
	HOP	A minimum of 15 feet of clear space	Ask student to hop 3 times, first on one foot and then on the other	1. Foot of nonsupport leg is bent and carried in back of the body 2. Nonsupport leg swings in pendular fashion to produce force ...

❐ The T.I.M.E. Toddler and Infant Motor Evaluation

AUTHORS: Lucy Jane Miller, PhD, OTR and Gale H. Roid, PhD

FORMAT: Rating scales based on observation of performance and optional interview.

PURPOSE: The T.I.M.E. provides a comprehensive and highly sensitive assessment of motor abilities and, more specifically, quality of movement in children. It is intended to identify motor delays or deviations, suggest appropriate remediation techniques, and examine the effectiveness of treatment. In addition, it defines theoretical constructs underlying motor development and links motor abilities to function.

POPULATION: Children ages 4 months to 3 1/2 years. (Standardization sample consisted of 731 children with and without motor delays or deviations and representing all test age ranges and the demographic distribution of the U.S. census.)

SETTING OR POSITION: A familiar private, distraction-free, warm area with a carpet or floor mat is preferable. Ventilation, light, and size of area must be adequate to accommodate the gross motor test, which involves spontaneous or elicited movements in the supine, prone, sitting, quadruped, and standing positions. The child should wear unrestrictive clothing that allows the examiner to observe movements. Specific preparations of materials are described.

MATERIALS OR TOOLS: The kit contains manual, record form booklets, timer, small toys, and containers. Examiner supplies masking tape, Cheerios, pens, pencils, and clipboard for scoring, and blanket if needed for the floor surface.

METHOD: T.I.M.E. consists of five primary subtests: Mobility, Stability, Motor Organization, Social/Emotional Abilities, and Functional Performance. Three additional clinical subtests for advanced analysis and research are: Quality Rating, Component Analysis, and Atypical Positions (these require advanced training or clinical expertise to administer). The examiner prompts the parent or caregiver to elicit specific motor abilities from the child, observing and recording scores during a 10–40 minute play period. Most subtests are designed for all test ages, although several subtests are administered at the child's specific developmental level. Some observations are timed. The Functional Performance Subtest is a recommended optional interview that gives information about the child's abilities in self-care, interactions, and functioning in the community; it requires an additional 15 minutes to administer and score. Scores for the various subtests are expressed in ratings, levels (i.e., maturity) achieved, or pass/fail checklist. The five primary subtests yield standard scaled scores, with tables for percentile scores and other statistical conversions (z-scores, stanines). Two clinical subtests yield only raw scores for clinical observations.

INTERPRETATION: A color classification system of final scores uses cut-off scores to indicate absence or presence of moderate or significant motor delays. In addition to quantitative scores, interpretation may be based on qualitative observation. The Component Analysis and Quality Rating subtests are optional for diagnostic purposes, treatment planning, and to measure effectiveness of intervention as they are sensitive to small increments of change. Motor Organization yields an additional growth score to compare the child's own changes in performance. The Functional Performance Subtest is important for showing how the child's mobility and stability affect quality of life.

RELIABILITY: Internal consistency estimates among subtests and by age groups ranged from .72–.97, most above .86. Test–retest reliability on a sample of 33 children with a 1- to 3-week interval were extremely high

(.97–.99). These data were used to determine the decision consistency for identifying children with motor delays: cut-off scores were highly reliable (.85–1.0). Interrater reliability, in which two examiners rated each of 31 children simultaneously, was .90 or higher (most near .99).

VALIDITY: Pediatric occupational therapy experts reviewed the literature, designed the initial items for measuring motor behavior, and field tested them with children. All items were analyzed to confirm that they were sufficiently sensitive to age, represented all levels of ability (Rasch analysis), discriminated between both groups (with and without motor delays), did not demonstrate racial bias, and fit into their subtest classification adequately (factor analysis).

SOURCE: Published by: Therapy Skill Builders, a division of Psychological Corporation, 555 Academic Court, San Antonio, TX 78204-2498. Tel: 800-228-0752; Fax: 800-232-1223. (**1994**)

COST: $$

SAMPLE: MOTOR ORGANIZATION   Circle all that apply.

throws 2 feet	throws 3 feet...	catches 2 feet...	tiptoes ≥ 2	steps 2x...	strings 1 cube

Cognitive

Assessments

❏ Allen Cognitive Level Test (ACL)

AUTHOR: Claudia Kay Allen, MA, OTR, FAOTA

FORMAT: Task analysis with standard demonstration-instruction.

PURPOSE: A routine task involving tool use is used to examine cognitive function in accordance with the author's theoretical hierarchy of cognitive levels of function. It is a clinical instrument to assess cognitive disability and suggest treatment approach.

POPULATION: Any psychiatric or cognitively impaired population; larger ACL is suitable for the elderly or visually impaired.

SETTING OR POSITION: Subject and examiner sit side-by-side at a slight angle in a distraction-free area with adequate lighting.

MATERIALS OR TOOLS: Kit includes leather pattern (regular or large size), leather laces, needles, and thread; in addition, needle-nose pliers are required.

METHOD: The ACL is available in the regular leather lace kit or the larger leather pattern. The examiner demonstrates and instructs subject in the leather-lacing stitch, following which the subject attempts two complete stitches. If successful, examiner repeats the steps with increasingly complex stitches (three in all). The subject is scored on the appropriate Cognitive Level (1–6) according to completion of stitches and methodology described by author. Additional comments on performance are noted by examiner.

INTERPRETATION: The assigned Cognitive Level indicates the level of cognitive function at which the subject can be expected to perform. The author further elaborates on the meaning and general functioning indicated by each of the levels.

RELIABILITY: Interrater reliability is .99.

VALIDITY: Content validity based on author's theory of cognitive levels; concurrent, construct, and possibly predictive validity are described, discriminating among schizophrenic, depressed, and nonpatient populations.

SOURCES: Obtain kit from: S&S Worldwide, PO Box 513, Colchester, CT 06415-0513. Tel: 800-243-9232; Fax: 800-566-6678.

Allen, C.K. (1982). Independence through activity: The practice of occupational therapy (psychiatry). *American Journal of Occupational Therapy, 36*(11), 731–739.

Allen, C.K., (1985). *Occupational therapy for psychiatric diseases: Measurement and management of cognitive disabilities.* Boston: Little, Brown.

COST: ¢; $ for Larger ACL (see Allen Diagnostic Module for more information).

SAMPLE: Level 2—Unable to imitate the running stitch. Level 3—Able to imitate the running stitch, two stitches.

❑ Allen Diagnostic Module (ADM)

AUTHOR: Catherine A. Earhart, OTR, Claudia Kay Allen, MA, OTR, FAOTA, and Tina Blue, OTR

FORMAT: Rating scale based on task performance.

PURPOSE: Standardized craft activities are used for the evaluation and treatment of individuals with cognitive disabilities. They provide a fast and inexpensive method of assessing the ability to process new information. The evaluation is based on Allen's theory of cognitive levels, with which the administrator must be familiar.

POPULATION: Adolescents and adults of both sexes who are at cognitive level 3.0 (attention to manual actions) and above. Use with chilren requires further investigation. Adaptations for physically disabled are offered.

SETTING OR POSITION: Individual and/or group set-up procedures are described in the manual for each activity, including storage and laying out of supplies and demonstration by therapist. (Group administration is permitted at cognitive levels 3.6 to 4.6.) Room should be well-lit without excessive noise or visual stimuli.

MATERIALS OR TOOLS: Manual, craft project kits including a completed demonstration sample, additional common supplies as indicated for each project (e.g., glue, scissors, pencil); ACL documentation computer software also is available.

METHOD: Twenty-four craft projects have been analyzed according to the complexity of cognitive skill required to perform them. Skills range from Allen's levels 3.0 to 5.8. Subject should be interviewed, observed, and tested with the Allen Cognitive Level Test (ACL) to determine appropriate level of evaluation on the ADM. Then a project is selected from the ADM repertoire. Manual contains a description for each project including: supplies, task instructions, indica-tions, set-up, therapist instructions, observations, and rating criteria. Adaptive techniques and equipment are suggested to accommodate physically disabled subjects. Length of assessment varies with the complexity of the project, ranging from 15 to 30 minutes to several days.

INTERPRETATION: The outcome, as determined by the rating sheet and observations, is expressed by numeral up to the maximum of 6.0, indicating the functional cognitive level. Further discussion of the cognitive levels describes the general capabilities of a subject at any given level. Computer software is available for documentation and generating reports.

RELIABILITY: The ADM is standardized in materials, instructions, and actions. Research is ongoing; certification and training conferences are available through S&S.

VALIDITY: Content and construct validity are described in Allen's earlier work on cognitive levels (see ACL). The ADM relies on single case method combined with professional judgment that is based on experience with and knowledge of cognitive levels and craft performance.

SOURCES: For instruction manual and crafts: S&S Worldwide, PO Box 513, Colchester, CT 06415-0513. Tel: 800-243-9232; Fax: 800-566-6678. (**1993**)

Allen, C.K., Earhart, C.A., & Blue, T. (1996). *Understanding cognitive performance modes.* Colchester, CT: S&S Worldwide.

COST: Manual—$$; Craft Kits—range: ¢–$$; Starter Kits—range: $$–$$$; Software—$$$; Handbook—$.

SAMPLE: Needlepoint Heart Key Ring (4.6–5.4)
    4.8 Attempts to attach ring but may need assistance.
    5.0 May attach ring without assistance.

❒ The Autobiographical Memory Interview (AMI)

AUTHORS: Michael Kopelman, Barbara Wilson, PhD, and Alan Baddeley

FORMAT: Semi-structured interview schedule.

PURPOSE: The value of assesssing autobiographical memory (the capacity to recollect facts and incidents from one's own life) using the AMI is, the authors propose, to help understand the nature of any memory deficit, to assist in intervention, to individualize subsequent management, and to facilitate research investigating anterograde versus retrograde amnesia.

POPULATION: Adults, from 18 years and up, including those with clinical disorders such as organic amnesic syndromes, dementia, and some psychiatric disorders. (Sample included 34 healthy control subjects and 62 amnesic patients at three hospitals in England.)

SETTING OR POSITION: The subject is seated comfortably in a quiet room. The examiner is seated with the scoresheet at a desk directly opposite the subject.

MATERIALS OR TOOLS: AMI manual, scoresheet, and pencil. A tape recorder may be used to record the interview with the subject's permission.

METHOD: The interview consists of two component parts assessing subject's past memories : the "personal semantic" schedule assesses recall of personal facts, and the "autobiographical incidents" schedule assesses recall of specific events. Both components address three broad time bands: childhood, early adult life, and recent facts/events. In the personal semantic section, the examiner asks specific questions; each response is scored by a point system for incorrect (0), partially correct (1/2 or 1), or correct (1 or 2) for a total of 21 possible points in each time band. The autobiographical incidents are prompted by a question, and responses are graded from 0–3 points depending on the degree of detail remem-

bered about each event, for a total of 9 points in each of the three time bands. Responses are recorded verbatim on the scoresheet. Memories can be verified by other informants, records, or by noting inconsistencies in the responses. The test is simple, quick to administer, and enjoyable and interesting to the subject.

INTERPRETATION: Cut-off scores based on the performance of healthy control subjects were set for "acceptable range," "borderline," "probably abnormal," and "definitely abnormal" in each component, each time band, and for test totals.

RELIABILITY: Test–retest reliability was determined by three raters independently scoring written descriptions of memories recalled; correlations between pairs of raters ranged from .83 to .86.

VALIDITY: Concurrent and construct validity were determined by several methods. AMI scores successfully discriminated amnesic patients from healthy control subjects. Intercorrelations between different remote memory test scores indicated that normal subjects who remember public information do not necessarily remember personal information, yet in spite of differences in types of remote memory, all remote memory tests correlated highly in the combined sample of healthy controls and patients. The intercorrelation between the two AMI components is high in both patient samples (.60 and .77). AMI supports evidence that some patients show a graded disruption in recent retrograde memories. Finally, the rate of inaccuracies of autobiographical memories among patients is generally very low.

SOURCE: Published by Thames Valley Test Company, Suffolk, England. Distributed in North America by: National Rehabilitation Services, 117 North Elm Street, PO Box 1247, Gaylord, MI 49735. Tel: 517-732-3866; Fax: 517-732-6164 (**1990**)

COST: $$

SAMPLE: Personal semantic questions

Ask for the subject's age when starting
at this school.

1 point for age

Autobiographic incident question

Ask the subject to recall an incident which
occurred while he or she was at primary school.

❏ Bay Area Functional Performance Evaluation (Second Edition) (BaFPE)

AUTHORS: Susan Lang Williams, MA, OTR, ATR and Judith Bloomer, MSW, OTR

FORMAT: Standardized task performance ratings and social observation scale.

PURPOSE: The tool assesses cognitive, affective, and performance skills in selected daily living tasks and social interaction skills. The results are intended to reflect the individual's level of function, as well as indicating community function and evaluating the effectiveness of occupational therapy.

POPULATION: The instrument was designed for the psychiatric population and is recommended for neurologically and mentally retarded populations. (Original sample consisted of 62 patients and 20 nonpatients ranging in age from 17 to 71 years; revised edition used 91 patients with acute psychotic disorder.)

SETTING OR POSITION: TOA—seated in well-lit, distraction-free environment with clock in view; SIS—two situations: one more and one less structured.

MATERIALS OR TOOLS: BaFPE Kit includes all materials and scoring sheets and a separate set of verbal instructions for the TOA.

METHOD: BaFPE consists of two subtests, the Task-Oriented Assessment (TOA) and the Social Interaction Scale (SIS), which can be administered independently or together. TOA: The subject is asked to complete five time-limited tasks and is rated on each, according to 12 well-defined behavioral guidelines, as well as observations specific to each task. The TOA is administered individually, requiring approximately 30–45 minutes.

SIS: A rater familiar with the subject observes the subject's social behavior in five defined situations. Based on clinical judgment, the rater assigns a score along a defined continuum in each of seven categories of social interaction. An optional self-report is included.

INTERPRETATION: TOA yields 3 component, 12 parameter, and 5 task scores, followed by a screening device for organic impairment. Preliminary norms are offered for comparison. SIS yields 5 situation, 7 parameter, and a total SIS score. In the absence of norms, a descriptive summary of social functioning is suggested. Parameter and component scores indicate areas of strength and weakness.

RELIABILITY: Interrater reliablility for TOA total score and performance components exceeded .90; cognitive components also exceeded .90 in three out of four test groups; and affective components (most subjective) ranged from .72 to .96 in four test groups. Task score correlations are also generally high (over .90). SIS correlations are lower, averaging .76 to .79 in two test groups.

VALIDITY: Content validity is based on compatibility of the instrument with several frames of reference in occupational therapy (e.g., Mosey, Riley) and most notably the model of human occupation. The original version of the BaFPE correlated with scores on the Functional Life Scale and the Global Assessment Scale, and it differentiated between psychotic and non-psychotic populations.

SOURCES: Published by: Maddak, Inc., 6 Industrial Road, Pequannock, NJ 07440. Tel: 800-443-4926; Fax: 201-305-0841. **(1978, revised 1987)**

Houston, D., Williams, S.L., Bloomer, J., & Mann, W.C. (1989). The Bay Area Functional Performance Evaluation: Development and standardization. *American Journal of Occupational Therapy, 43*(3), 170.

Bloomer, J., & Williams, S.K., (1982). The Bay Area

Functional Performance Evaluation. In B. Hemphill (Ed.), *The evaluative process in psychiatric occupational therapy* (pp. 255–308). Thorofare, NJ: Slack.

COST: $$$

SAMPLE: TOA: "I would like you to sort these shells so that you put all the shells that are similar in size, shape and color into the same container."

SIS: Response to Authority Figures —(ranges from) not able to assess due to degree of dysfunction —(to) almost always appropriate interaction with, or response to, authority figures.

◻ Blessed Dementia Rating Scale

AUTHORS: G. Blessed, B.E. Tomlinson, and Martin Roth

FORMAT: Rating scale and checklist based on semi-structured interview and mental tasks.

PURPOSE: The Dementia Rating Scale attempts to quantify the degree of intellectual and personality deterioration in people with dementia, based on their ability to deal with the practical tasks of everyday life as well as on simple psychological tests.

POPULATION: Elderly people with dementia. (Sample consisted of 264 patients admitted to a psychiatric hospital, a geriatric hospital, and a selected ward of a general hospital.)

SETTING OR POSITION: Not prescribed.

MATERIALS OR TOOLS: Dementia scale and pencil.

METHOD: The scale consists of 22 items relating to competence in personal, domestic, and social activities. Information is obtained by questioning a close friend or relative about the subject's performance in daily living tasks during the preceding 6 months. Each item is then scored 1 (total incompetence), 1/2 (partial or intermittent incapacity), or 0 (fully preserved), or given points (0–3) according to stated criteria for changes in habits or personality.

INTERPRETATION: Total score ranges from 0, reflecting fully preserved capacity, to 28, which reflects extreme incapacity.

RELIABILITY: Not discussed.

VALIDITY: Test scores differentiated between patients with senile dementia registering poor mean scores and other medical and psychiatric patient groups. Post-mortem investigation of 60 patients revealed highly significant correlations (-.591) between test scores and cerebral plaque counts.

SOURCE: Blessed, G., Tomlinson, B.E., Roth, M. The association between quantitative measures of dementia and of senile change in the cerebral grey matter of elderly subjects. *British Journal of Psychiatry, 114,* 797–811. (**1968**)

COST: ¢

SAMPLE: Changes in Performance of Everyday Activities

Inability to cope with small sums of money	1	1/2	0
Tendency to dwell in the past	1	1/2	0

❐ Clinical Dementia Rating (CDR)

AUTHOR: John C. Morris, MD

FORMAT: Rating scale based on semistructured interview.

PURPOSE: The CDR is designed to measure and follow the natural history (i.e., irrespective of intervention) of senile dementia of the Alzheimer's type (SDAT). It provides a classification system for describing stages of severity of the disease for clinical as well as research purposes.

POPULATION: Adults with SDAT. (Sample consisted of 25 subjects from the Memory and Aging Project at Washington University, St. Louis.)

SETTING OR POSITION: Not prescribed.

MATERIALS OR TOOLS: CDR and pencil.

METHOD: The CDR consists of six categories ("boxes") of cognitive function commonly affected in SDAT: memory, orientation, judgment and problem solving, involvement in community affairs, involvement at home and in hobbies, and personal care. Subjects and their informants are interviewed using the Initial Subject Protocol, a semistructured clinical interview that takes about 90 minutes to administer. From this information, the six box scores are independently rated on a 5-point scale according to descriptions of impairment. These scores are averaged according to instructions to obtain the Clinical Dementia Rating.

INTERPRETATION: The overall CDR describes the subject along with a 5-point scale as: without dementia (0), or with questionable (0.5), mild (1), moderate (2), or severe (3) dementia.

RELIABILITY: Videotaped interviews of 25 subjects were each rated by two clinicians to determine interrater reliability of .90 on the overall CDR and ranging from .68 to .88 on the individual category ratings. The reliability of the individual ratings were determined by correlating the sums of the box scores: 76% within one point of each other, 88% within two, and 100% of the box sums were within three points of each other.

VALIDITY: The CDR was validated against postmortem examinations of 2 subjects who were normal and 26 subjects with SDAT, demonstrating that all ratings were verified in every stage of the disease.

SOURCES: Obtain from John C. Morris, MD, Memory and Aging Project, Washington University School of Medicine, 660 South Euclid Avenue, PO Box 8111, St. Louis, MO 63110. Tel: 314-362-2683.

Published in: Morris, J.C. (1993). The Clinical Dementia Rating (CDR): Current version and scoring rules. *Neurology, 43*(11), 2,412–2,414.

Burke, W.J., Miller, P., Rubin, E.H., Morris, J.C., Coben, L.A., Duchek, J., Wittels, I.G., & Berg, L. (1988). Reliability of the Washington University Clinical Dementia Rating. *Archives of Neurology, 45*, 31–32.

COST: ¢

SAMPLE: Home and Hobbies

None (0)—Life at home, hobbies, and intellectual interests well maintained.

Moderate (2)—Only simple chores preserved; very restricted interests, poorly maintained.

❏ Cognitive Adaptive Skills Evaluation (CASE)

AUTHORS: G. N. Masagatani, Ed., OTR, MEd, FAOTA, C. S. Nielson, OTR, and E. R. Ranslow, OTR

FORMAT: Skills inventory using interview, observation, and task performance.

PURPOSE: The tool is designed to examine an individual's cognitive process while performing a task. It is intended to survey functional skills, using the theories of Piaget, Mosey, Singer, and Allen.

POPULATION: Developed for use with psychiatric patients, but applicable to adults and adolescents with cognitive disorders.

SETTING OR POSITION: Work table with materials laid out in front of subject.

MATERIALS OR TOOLS: Prescribed writing implements and paper, ruler, sample calendar, written directions, protocol sheet, evaluation summary sheet, and pencil needed by examiner.

METHOD: The subject is asked to perform a task (making a calendar) and respond to interview questions related to the task. Then the subject repeats the task and responds to a second set of interview questions related to both tasks. The examiner records the behaviors on the protocol sheet based on observations of the performance and on subject's responses. Results are summarized and analyzed according to defined behavioral criteria. These can be discussed with the subject for confirmation. The method yields performance summaries stated in behavioral terms. The entire process requires 45–60 minutes.

RELIABILITY: Authors report high interrater reliability; examiners are advised to familiarize themselves with the theories of Piaget and Mosey before administering CASE.

VALIDITY: Content validity is demonstrated by research on the theories of Piaget and Mosey, and by trial administration to identify behaviors.

SOURCES: Obtain from: Gladys Masagatani, Eastern Kentucky University, Department of Occupational Therapy, Dizney 103, Richmond, KY 40475-3135. Tel: 606-622-3300. (**1979; revised 1994**)

Hemphill, B. (publication pending 1996). *Integrative process.* Thorofare, NJ: Slack.

Masagatani, G., et al. (1981). *Cognitive adaptive skills evaluation manual.* New York: Haworth Press.

COST: $

SAMPLE: "Do you understand what I mean by a calendar for a week?"

"Can you tell me how to make one?"

❒ Cognitive Assessment of Minnesota (CAM)

AUTHORS: Ruth A. Rustad, OTR, Terry L. DeGroot, OTR, Margaret L. Jungkunz, OTR, Karen S. Freeberg, OTR, Laureen G. Borowick, OTR, and Ann M. Wanttie, OTR

FORMAT: Screening test using question-and-answer and performance tasks.

PURPOSE: This test provides a concise hierarchical approach to screening a wide range of cognitive skills in order to identify general problem areas and guide the selection of specific treatment activities. It can be used as a baseline of the individual's deficits and abilities, to measure change, and to indicate areas for in-depth investigation.

POPULATION: Adults who have sustained a brain injury or cerebrovascular accident (CVA) and who are at Level IV and above on the Rancho Los Amigos Cognitive Scale. (Normative sample consisted of 200 subjects, ages 18 to 70, without impairment or neurological history.)

SETTING OR POSITION: Bedside or clinic with few distractions, examiner sitting directly opposite subject at a table or writing surface.

MATERIALS OR TOOLS: Included in the carrying portfolio are the manual, laminated test cards, and score booklets; in addition, paper, tape, coins, cubes, ruler, scissors, timer, pencil, and a list of common objects are needed.

METHOD: CAM consists of 17 subtests ranging from simple to complex and covering a wide variety of abilities, such as attention, memory, visual neglect, math, ability to follow directions, and judgment. They are arranged according to a theoretical hierarchy of four levels of cognitive skills needed to accomplish a task: fund of knowledge, manipulation of old knowledge, social awareness and judgment, and abstract thinking. CAM may be administered in one or two sessions to avoid fatigue. For each subtest, written instructions and scoring procedures are provided in addition to purpose, materials, administration, and areas to rule out (e.g., sensory or perceptual deficits). Raw subtest scores are combined for a total CAM score of 0–80. The test requires approximately 40 minutes.

INTERPRETATION: The raw scores are plotted on a scoring profile, organized by the cognitive hierarchy. The scores are graphed to illustrate scoring categories of: None to Mild (deficit), Moderate, and Severe.

RELIABILITY: Internal consistency by inter-item analysis indicated all items measure the same construct. Interrater reliability for 39 impaired subjects scored by two raters simultaneously showed statistically significant agreement on all items as well as on the total score (.94). Test–retest reliability with impaired and nonimpaired subjects over a 1-week interval demonstrated consistent total scale score (.96), although total score of CVA group increased slightly.

VALIDITY: Items were selected by occupational therapists experienced in cognitive rehabilitation. Total CAM score discriminated between 95% of impaired and nonimpaired subjects, establishing a cut-off score for probable impairment. Concurrent validity is supported by agreement of total CAM scores with clinical appraisal of cognitive skills and with scores on the Porteus Maze Test and Mini-Mental Status Exam in the impaired population.

SOURCE: Published by: Therapy Skill Builders, a division of The Psychological Corporation, 555 Academic Court, San Antonio, TX 78204-2498. Tel: 800-228-0752; Fax: 800-232-1223. (**1993**)

COST: $$

SAMPLE: Following Directions
a. Appropriate Yes/No
"Nod your head yes."
"Shake your head no." ...
b. One-step verbal directions
"Shut your eyes." ...

❏ Cognitive Performance Test (CPT)

AUTHOR: Theressa Burns, OTR

FORMAT: Standardized graded task performance.

PURPOSE: CPT is a functional assessment of ADL tasks requiring information processing skills. Based on early Allen Cognitive Level Theory, it determines the degree to which cognitive processing deficits compromise performance of common activities. It is useful in research and clinical assessment to predict functional capabilities in various contexts.

POPULATION: Adults with Alzheimer's disease (AD). (Sample is based on 77 patients with mild to moderate AD and 15 normal elderly control subjects at a geriatric research center in Minneapolis.)

SETTING OR POSITION: The standardized set-up for each task is described, as is position of subject as necessary.

MATERIALS OR TOOLS: Materials are specified for each task, requiring pertinent common items (e.g., wardrobe or rack with specific items of clothing arranged on it for the dressing task).

METHOD: CPT consists of six tasks (Dress, Shop, Toast, Phone, Wash, and Travel), each given standard equipment, set-up, and method of administration. The subject is asked to perform each task, with verbal reassurance, cuing, directions, or demonstration as needed. If difficulty with performance is observed, contingency directions allow for adding or eliminating sensory cues as needed. Graded scoring guidelines are provided for each task.

INTERPRETATION: Scores range from Level 1 (lowest) to 6 on each task. Total test score ranges from 6–33 and represents average task performance when divided by 6. CPT results may be generalized to capabilities and needs of the subject in all but very complex tasks of daily living. Based on early Allen research, persons functioning at level 5 may be expected to live independently with some support, and so on for the other levels. Treatment planning may be based on the type of difficulty demonstrated.

RELIABILITY: Interrater reliability between two testers is .91; test–retest reliability with a 4-week interval is .89. Internal consistency of the CPT is .84.

VALIDITY: Construct validity is demonstrated by significant correlations between CPT scores and Mini-Mental State Examination scores (.67) and two ADL measures rated by caregivers (Instrumental ADL .64 and Physical Self-Maintenance Scale .49). Predicitive validity identified risk of institutionalization with the progression of the disease over each of 3 years of follow-up, and time of institutionalization for low scorers was 624 days versus 1,294 days for high scorers. CPT also discriminated between normal subjects and those with AD.

SOURCES: Published in: Allen, C. K., Earhart, C. A., & Blue, T. *Occupational therapy treatment goals for the physically and cognitively disabled.* Bethesda, MD: American Occupational Therapy Association. **(1992)**

Burns, T., Mortimer, J.A., & Merchak, P. (1994). Cognitive Performance Test: A new approach to functional assessment in Alzheimer's Disease. *Journal of Geriatric Psychiatry and Neurology, 7,* 46–54.

COST: ¢

SAMPLE: Dress: ..."I want you to get dressed as if you were going outside on a cold, rainy day...Would you take anything else from the closet?"

❑ Contextual Memory Test (CMT)

AUTHOR: Joan P. Toglia, MA, OTR

FORMAT: Verbal questionnaire and performance task.

PURPOSE: The Contextual Memory Test was designed to assess awareness of memory capacity, use of strategy, and recall in adults with memory dysfunction. It can be used as a screen to determine the need for further evaluation or to indicate how responsive the individual is to memory cues, thereby recommending compensatory or remedial treatment.

POPULATION: Adults age 18 years and older who have neurological or organic memory impairment and are able to follow two-step directions, recognize objects, and communicate; the test has been used with psychiatric patients and may be useful with older children and adolescents, but studies have not been completed with these populations. (Normative sample is based on 375 adults, ages 17–86, most from New York City area.)

SETTING OR POSITION: Quiet room with adequate lighting and no distractions.

MATERIALS OR TOOLS: Kit includes carrying folder with manual, two picture cards each containing 20 individual drawings related to a theme, two sets of 40 recognition cards (pictures of individual items), and scoring booklet; plus pencil and stopwatch.

METHOD: CMT contains a memory questionnaire about the subject's memory capabilities and strategies, plus a memory task. It is hypothesized that using meaningful objects will better relate to memory skills needed in everyday function. Thus the memory task uses pictures of related objects on a theme: a restaurant and a morning routine. The picture card is shown for 90 seconds after which the subject is asked to recall as many items in it as possible. The delayed recall task requires the same item recall, after doing another activity. during a 15–20 minute interval. Following delayed recall, the subject is asked questions regarding awareness of performance. If performance is below the norm, the subject is given information on the context of the pictures to determine the benefit of cues. (The subject may indicate responses using recognition cards instead of verbal recall if necessary.) Scores are based on the number of correct responses. Administration requires 5–10 minutes, in addition to the 15- to 20-minute delayed task. Two equivalent forms of the test allow retesting to monitor change.

INTERPRETATION: The test yields three recall scores (immediate, delayed, and total), and scores for cued recall, recognition, awareness, and strategy use. Scores are compared to the norms and then analyzed for patterns using the Summary of Findings worksheet. Recall scores are classified into categories of WNL (within normal limits), suspect, mild, moderate, or severe deficit. The author suggests methods of interpreting score discrepancies in each area and offers guidelines for treatment.

RELIABILITY: Analysis of item and test equivalence allowed the development of standard scores to account for differences in difficulty. Parallel form reliability (second version given 3–36 hours later) ranged from .73–.81, with prediction scores (subject predicted own score) correlating at .90 and strategy scores at .75. Test–retest reliability was estimated by comparing immediate recall with delayed recall scores (control subjects .74–.87, brain injured .85–.94). Rasch analysis supports item separation reliability (item spread is discernible, with a .92–.96 range among tests) and person separation (.75–.80). Interrater reliability studies are in progress.

VALIDITY: Concurrent validity was demonstrated by .80–.84 correlations with specified Rivermead Behavioral Memory Test scores. Rasch analysis indicated the item difficulties are better suited to brain-injured than control subjects. Scores discriminated between nondisabled and brain-injured subjects.

SOURCE: Published by: Therapy Skill Builders, a division of The Psychological Corporation, 555 Academic Court, San Antonio, TX 78204-2498. Tel: 800-228-0752; Fax: 800-232-1223. **(1993)**

COST: $$

SAMPLE: Questionnaire

If you studied 20 objects for half a minute, how many do you think you would be able to remember?_____

Would you remember facts about this form a week from now? (Circle one.) |1| No |2| Yes

❒ Doors and People

AUTHORS: Alan Baddeley, Hazel Emslie, and Ian Nimmo-Smith

FORMAT: Norm-based performance test.

PURPOSE: This test of visual and verbal recall and recognition was designed to isolate these abilities from other skills, such as perception and copying, common to many memory tests. It is sensitive to a wide range of memory capabilities (subtle to severe), and the tasks are acceptable to mature populations.

POPULATION: Adults, applicable to a wide range of subject groups and diagnoses. (Norms are based on a stratified sample consisting of 238 subjects divided among 6 social class categories and 5 age bands ranging from 16–97 years.)

SETTING OR POSITION: Subject and examiner presumed to be seated at a table in a distraction-free room.

MATERIALS OR TOOLS: Kit includes manual, scoresheets, stimulus cards; and a pencil and paper.

METHOD: The test consists of four subtests: the Doors Test (visual recognition), the Shapes Test (visual recall), the Names Test (verbal recognition), and the People Test (verbal recall).

The Doors Test consists of colored photographs of "target doors" mounted singly and then presented with distractor doors for each recognition set; the subject will be shown 12 target doors and then asked to recognize them on the distractor sheets (two sets are included, easy and difficult).

The Shapes Test contains four distinct line drawings of crosses selected because they are easy to draw; after copying each from the master drawing, the subject is asked to draw them from memory (immediately and again after a delay).

The Names Test uses target forename/surname pairs mounted singly and then presented with distractor names that share the same forename (selected from common English and Scottish names); the subject is asked to read each target name aloud and then recognize them on the distractor sheets.

The People Test consists of three common and one uncommon forename/surname pair combined with an occupation (e.g., doctor, minister), and each presented as a caption to a color photograph of the character; the subject reads each name aloud from the photograph and must recall the four names afterward (immediate and delayed). Occupation and photograph serve as memory aids.

One point is given for each correct item (1 point each for forename, surname, and correct pairing on the People Test), except for the Shapes Test in which each drawing receives up to 3 points, according to written criteria.

INTERPRETATION: The overall memory scaled score is the most reliable and sensitive index of episodic memory performance. Subscores can be used to contrast verbal and visual scores or recall and recognition, although with lower reliability so that deficits observed should be tested further. A forgetting score may be calculated from the raw data based on the difference between the learning trials and delayed recall scores.

RELIABILITY: Information is not available in the manual.

VALIDITY: The test has been shown to be sensitive to a variety of diagnostic groups, including Alzheimer's disease, stroke, normal ageing, and schizophrenia, as well as for comparison of right and left temporal lobe surgery. There is preliminary evidence that different etiologies result in different patterns of memory deficits, as evident in subtest scores.

SOURCE: Published by Thames Valley Test Company, Suffolk, England. Distributed in North America by: National Rehabilitation Services, 117 North Elm Street, PO Box 1247, Gaylord, Michigan 49735. Tel: 517-732-3866; Fax: 517-732-6164. (1994)

COST: $$

SAMPLE: Verbal recall: the People Test
The tester turns over the first page of the People Test items and says:

> 'This is the doctor. His name is Jim Green'. ...
> 'This is the minister. His name is Cuthbert Cattermole'.

Repeat for the other two cards. After the fourth remove the cards and say:

> 'Now let's see if you can remember them. What was the doctor's name?... the minister's name?...' and so on.

☐ Global Deterioration Scale (GDS), including Brief Cognitive Rating Scale (BCRS) and Functional Assessment Staging (FAST)

AUTHORS: GDS: Barry Reisberg, MD, Steven H. Ferris, PhD, Mony J. De Leon, EdD, and Thomas Crook, PhD; BCRS and FAST: Barry Reisberg, MD, Steven G. Sclan, PhD, Emile Franssen, MD, Alan Kluger, PhD, and Steven Ferris, PhD

FORMAT: Behavior-based rating scales.

PURPOSE: The scales were developed to assess the clinically identifiable and ratable stages of primary degenerative dementia and age-associated memory impairment. They are used to describe and follow the onset and gradual progression of the disease and to communicate the level of cognitive and functional decline to others.

POPULATION: Patients with primary degenerative dementia. (GDS was developed over a 5-year period from thousands of patient interviews; BCRS and FAST were derived from GDS.)

SETTING OR POSITION: Not prescribed (should be administered before pharmacologic treatment).

MATERIALS OR TOOLS: Scale (additional psychometric measures are used to verify the rating).

METHOD: GDS consists of 7 well-defined stages, ranging from no cognitive decline to very severe cognitive decline. Each stage is described by clinical characteristics and by psychometric concomitants (using the Guild Memory Tests, WAIS vocabulary score, and the 10-question Mental Status Questionnaire). Based on observation and skilled clinical interview by trained personnel (e.g., psychiatrist), a rating is given indicating the stage of disease of the subject. Accurate rating of stages 1–7 is based on accurate clinical diagnosis of the syndrome by a trained professional, as well as on the description of clinical course and presentation.

For more detailed staging of severe Alzheimer's disease (AD), BCRS and the FAST were developed (Reisberg, et al., 1994). BCRS comprises clinical assessments corresponding to GDS (axis V), plus 4 axes of cognitive ability: (I) concentration, (II) recent memory, (III) remote memory, and (IV) orientation. FAST identifies 16 successive functional stages and substages of AD, with 11 substages corresponding to GDS stages 6–7 and reflecting severe impairment rarely distinguished by other assessments.

INTERPRETATION: While actual diagnosis may require training in psychiatric medicine, the rating systems are universally suitable in describing the cognitive skills and resulting activities of daily living (ADL) status of the subject over the long disease course.

RELIABILITY: Reliability studies (Reisberg, et al., 1994) summarized reliability coefficients ranging from .82 (test–retest; intraclass) to .92 (test–retest; interrater) and .92–.97 for interrater (between examiner and simultaneous observers) for a variety of diagnoses. BCRS studies found test–retest and interrater reliability to range from .76–.82 and .86 (test–retest/interrater) and .82–.97 (simultaneous interrater) for axes I–IV. FAST reliability is somewhat dependent on BCRS axis V (7 functional levels) from which it was derived. Other FAST reliability studies demonstrated coefficients of .86–.87 (intraclass), .76 and .96 (simultaneous interrater), and .83 (test–retest/interrater).

VALIDITY: Content validity is based on statistical analysis of the components of the 7 stages, and on agreement with the weighting of the description phrases by family members and clinicians (Reisberg, et al., 1994). The scale was also validated against behavioral, neuroanatomic, and neurophysiologic measures. In retrospective analysis of the relationship between scores and independent psychometric assessments, significant correlations were noted with the majority of measures. In addition, scores correlated with CT scans (.62 and .53) and PET scans (.69–.83) to demonstrate significant relationships with anatomic and metabolic brain changes (Reisberg, et al., 1982).

FAST scores correlated with independent psychometric test measures (.59–.73), clinical assessment (> 83–.94), and Mini-Mental State Examination scores (.87); these studies are limited by the bottoming out of most cognitive assessment measures (Reisberg, 1988). The ordinal pattern of functional deterioration of the FAST was also confirmed (.76) (Reisberg et al., 1994). Finally, correlations between FAST and adapted infant cognitive assessment, reflex responses (paratonia), and pathologic reflex release signs (grasp, sucking) are evident in stage 7 of impairment (Reisberg et al., 1994).

SOURCES: GDS and FAST published in: Reisberg, B., Sclan, S.G., Franssen, E., Kluger, A., & Ferris, S. Dementia staging in chronic care populations, *Alzheimer Disease and Associated Disorders*, *8*, suppl. 1, S188–S205. (**1994**)

BCRS published in: Reisberg, B., & Ferris, S. H. The Brief Cognitive Rating Scale (BCRS). *Psychopharmacology Bulletin*, *24*, 629–636. (**1988**)

Reisberg, B., Ferris, S.H., De Leon, M.J., & Crook, T. The Global Deterioration Scale for assessment of primary degenerative dementia. *American Journal of Psychiatry*, *139*, 1136–1139. (**1982**)

Reisberg, B. Functional Assessment Staging (FAST). *Psychopharmacology Bulletin*, *24*, 653–659.

Address reprint requests to: Dr. Barry Reisberg, MD, Department of Psychiatry, New York University Medical Center, 550 First Avenue, New York, NY 10016.

COST: ¢

SAMPLE: (GDS) *Stage 7: Very severe cognitive decline*

All verbal abilities are lost over the course of this stage.

Early in this stage words and phrases are spoken but speech is very circumscribed.

Later there is no speech at all—only grunting.

(FAST)

7a Speech ability limited to about a half-dozen words

 b Intelligible vocabulary limited to a single word

❑ Goodenough-Harris Drawing Test

AUTHORS: Florence L. Goodenough and Dale B. Harris

FORMAT: Standardized drawing test.

PURPOSE: The test, revised from the Goodenough Draw-a-Man Test, is designed as a nonverbal test of conceptual maturity, an indicator of intellectual ability. (Note: The authors caution that children's drawings reflect concepts that develop with experience and knowledge; this test should not be used to determine creativity, interests, or psychological conflicts.)

POPULATION: Children ages 3 to 15 years. (Norms are based on 2,975 children, ages 5 to 15, from geographic and socioeconomic distribution in the U.S.)

SETTING OR POSITION: Not prescribed.

MATERIALS OR TOOLS: Manual, test booklet, set of quality scale cards, pencil (no. 2 1/2 preferred).

METHOD: The child is asked to make three pencil drawings, one at a time: a man, a woman, and self. Each drawing is to be carefully executed and include the whole body. The test can be administered in groups, but if administered individually, it should be followed by an informal interview to clarify ambiguities in the pictures. The Man and Woman pictures may be scored according to carefully delineated point scales or according to quality scales for a quick estimate of the score. The point scales are based on the number of details present in the drawing, which are totaled for the raw score. The quality scales provide prescored sample pictures for rating the test drawings. The self drawing generally is not scored, as it is not standardized. The test usually is completed in 10 to 15 minutes.

INTERPRETATION: The raw score is converted to a standard score equivalent, which gives the child's standing relative to age and sex norms, or to a percentile rank.

RELIABILITY: Interrater reliability varies from low .80s to high .90s in numerous studies summarized. Test–retest reliability ranged from the .60s and .70s.

VALIDITY: Test scores are associated with intellectual maturity, as measured by the Stanford-Binet or WISC.

SOURCE: Test kit published by: Harcourt, Brace, Jovanovich, Inc., Psychological Corporation, 555 Academic Court, San Antonio, TX 78204-2498. Tel: 800-228-0752; Fax: 800-232-1223.

Manual reprinted from: Harris, D.B. (1963). *Children's drawings as measures of intellectual maturity: A revision and extension of the Goodenough Draw-a-Man Test.*

COST: $$

SAMPLE: "I want you to make a picture of a man. Make the very best picture that you can...be sure to make the whole man."

❑ Leiter International Performance Scale (revision pending)

[**NOTE:** This revision is still in the development phase, substantially changing the traditional form of the Leiter. As a result, the description contained here is a preliminary one based on discussion with the project manager. The instrument is included in this text because of its longstanding prominence and its increased application to occupational therapy.]

AUTHORS: Gale H. Roid, PhD and Lucy J. Miller, PhD, OTR/L

FORMAT: Norm-based performance scale.

PURPOSE: The Leiter was developed to provide a culture-free, nonverbal means of assessing general intelligence, based on primarily abstract concepts and using manipulative responses.

POPULATION: Individuals ages 2 years through adult. It is well-suited for those with motor impairments, speech or hearing impairments, cognitive delays, or who speak English as a second language, according to the project director for the new revision. (Normative sample of revised version includes 1,800 children, ages 2 through 20 years, and is based on 1994 U.S. census; over 700 children comprise delayed and disabled groups.)

SETTING OR POSITION: The test requires a table with examiner seated opposite the subject. New version uses a spiral binder of stimulus pictures placed upright in easel position, with front tray containing stalls for response cards facing the subject.

MATERIALS OR TOOLS: Handbook, report forms, and pencil for examiner. The new format will use spiral binder with response playing-type cards in place of the carrying case with trays and blocks.

METHOD: The Leiter consists of a Core Battery with two components (visualization and reasoning) and a

Supplemental Battery with two components (memory and attention). Each battery contains 10 subtests in which response cards are matched to the stimulus template pattern (previously blocks to frames) according to increasingly complex intellectual judgments. The subject is required to put the correct card (block) into the matching compartment by color, design, classification, series, etc. No verbal directions are given. Each item is scored as pass/fail by the number of blocks placed correctly. Administration of each battery requires 45–60 minutes.

INTERPRETATION: The Leiter yields scaled scores for each of the 20 subtests, domain scores for each of the four components, standard scores and percentiles. A global intelligence quotient score (previously included Mental Age) is calculated from the total results. The Leiter can be used to compare the subject to the norms, or to determine absolute improvement in the individual child over time according to cognitive growth scales.

RELIABILITY: Extensive reliability data have been described for the original version (internal consistency .75, test–retest .91 for mentally retarded sample, with a range of .36 for deaf preschoolers to .92 for aphasic children, using the Arthur Adaptation of the test materials). Research is now in progress for the new format.

VALIDITY: Correlations between the original Leiter and numerous other intelligence measures (Stanford-Binet .77, Wechsler .78, Peabody Picture Vocabulary .57, teacher ratings .76 intelligence and .60 achievement, and more) have been reported. The revision is currently undergoing Rasch analysis to develop the cognitive growth scales.

SOURCE: Published by: Stoelting Co., 620 Wheat Lane, Wood Dale, IL 60191. Tel: 800-860-9775; Fax: 708-860-

9775. (1927, revised 1948, 1979, and pending 1996–1997)

COST: $$$$; purchase is restricted to those trained or otherwise qualified.

SAMPLE: Instructions not yet available.

❒ Loewenstein Occupational Therapy Cognitive Assessment (LOTCA)

AUTHORS: Malka Itzkovich, OTR, Betty Elazar,OTR, Sarah Averbuch, MA, OTR, and Principal Researcher, Noomi Katz, PhD, OTR

FORMAT: Battery comprised of oral response and task performance ratings.

PURPOSE: This concise battery of qualitative, client-centered tests is designed for use by occupational therapists working in neurological rehabilitation. It is used to identify abilities and limitations in areas of cognitive processing, as a basis for treatment planning, and to evaluate change resulting from intervention.

POPULATION: Brain-injured patients, including diagnoses of traumatic head injury, cerebral vascular accidents, and tumors. (Two samples consisted of 48 brain-injured and 55 normal adults, and 240 normal children ages 6 to 12 years, in Israel; scores of 25 American subjects from a New England hospital and a long-term-care facility were compared.)

SETTING OR POSITION: Not prescribed, although several test procedures requiring subject to copy with paper and pencil or using objects spread in front of subject, assume subject to be seated at a table.

MATERIALS OR TOOLS: Test kit consists of manual and test booklet, blocks, scissors, comb, pencil, pegs and pegboard, test cards, shapes, puzzle, and envelope. A box of matches is needed.

METHOD: The battery consists of 20 subtests, including Riska Object Classification, or ROC. Four areas are assessed: orientation, perception, visuomotor organization, and thinking operations. For each test, materials, procedure, and scoring criteria are described in the manual (see Williams Riska & Allen [1985] for administration and scoring of ROC). Scores are based on a scale from 1 (low) to 4 (high), except for categorization tests,

which are scored from 1 to 5. Level of attention and concentration during testing are also rated. Space for comments is provided on the scoresheet. The battery takes 30–45 minutes and may be administered in 1 to 3 sessions. Procedures for aphasic patients are included.

INTERPRETATION: Results are recorded on the scoresheet, which provides a profile of performance, indicating areas of strength and weakness. Retesting allows comparison of scores to assess change. The sample of normal children offers mean performance scores to compare with subjects ages 6 to 12.

RELIABILITY: Interrater reliability among three raters ranged from .82–.97; six ratings of a single videotaped performance reached .86–1.00 agreement for all tests. Internal consistency for three of the test areas are: .87 for five perception tests, .95 for eight visuomotor organization tests, and .85 for five thinking operations tests.

VALIDITY: LOTCA was found to differentiate between the patient and control sample in all tests. The visuomotor organization tests correlate with the Wechsler Adult Intelligence Scale Block Design subtest (.68–.69 using standard procedure, and .77–.78 using untimed Block Design, in a brain-injured sample and a schizophrenic patient group respectively). Factor analysis was used to confirm that the 18 tests (excluding orientation) clustered into the three test areas; variability among factors is discussed.

SOURCE: Developed by: Lowenstein Rehabilitation Hospital, Israel. Published by: Maddak, Inc., 6 Industrial Road, Pequannock, NJ 07440. Tel: 800-443-4926; Fax: 201-305-0841. (**1990**)

For ROC, see: Williams Riska, L., & Allen, C.K. (1985). Research with non-disabled population. In C.K. Allen (Ed.), *Occupational therapy for psychiatric diseases: Measurement and management of cognitive disabilities,* (pp. 315–338). Boston: Little Brown.

Cermak, S.A., Katz, N., McGuire, E., Greenbaum, S., Peralta, C., & Maser-Flanagan, V. (1995). Performance of Americans and Israelis with cerebrovascular accident on the Loewenstein Occupational Therapy Cognitive Assessment (LOTCA). *American Journal of Occupational Therapy, 49*(6), 500–506.

COST: $$$

SAMPLE: Reproduction of a Puzzle

...."Construct the puzzle **on** the design."

1 Point—P. (patient) is unable to perform.

2 Points—P. is only able to put in the three central vertical pieces.

3 Points—P. performs with trial and error but achieves good performance.

4 Points—Good performance without trial and error.

❑ The Middlesex Elderly Assessment of Mental State (MEAMS)

AUTHOR: Evelyn Golding, PhD

FORMAT: Standard screening test using verbal and paper-and-pencil tasks

PURPOSE: MEAMS detects gross impairment of specific cognitive skills in the elderly. By systematically surveying functions from different areas of the brain, it is designed to differentiate between functional illnesses and organically based cognitive impairments, and to determine which areas of the brain are functioning less efficiently.

POPULATION: Elderly. (Sample consisted of 120 patients of a day hospital in London, ages 65 to 93.)

SETTING OR POSITION: Subject is seated opposite the examiner with the flip chart standing or laid flat between them.

MATERIALS OR TOOLS: Kit includes test manual, flip charts with instructions and picture cards, score sheet, pencil.

METHOD: MEAMS consists of 12 subtests, each requiring the subject to perform a simple cognitive task (e.g., identify an object in an unconventional photograph, learn a name, identify an item by its verbal description). The examiner flips the pages of the flip chart, following the instructions printed on the pages facing the examiner while exhibiting the stimulus pages in sequence to the subject. Each subtest response is scored as pass (1) or fail (0), and all scores are added up for a total MEAMS score (maximum=12). Two parallel versions of the MEAMS flip chart allows for reassessment with an equivalent instrument. The test can be completed in approximately 10 minutes.

INTERPRETATION: The author suggests the following guidelines based on the validation study: scores 10–12 are within normal range, 8–9 is borderline and factors of intelligence and the physical and emotional state of the subject should be considered, and below 7 indicates the need for a full cognitive evaluation. Since all items should be passed by normal elderly subjects regardless of intelligence, failing scores indicate areas of likely cognitive impairment.

RELIABILITY: High interrater reliability (.98) was determined by separate but simultaneous scoring of two raters. The correlation between the two parallel forms of the test was .91.

VALIDITY: Construct validity was demonstrated by statistically significant differences in subtest scores between subjects diagnosed with dementia and those diagnosed with depression without dementia. The mini-memory test was not included in the original validation study, but was later found to distinguish between subjects with Azheimer's disease and depressed patients without dementia, and it correlated well with total screening test scores.

SOURCE: Published by Thames Valley Test Company, Suffolk, England. Distributed in North America by: National Rehabilitation Services, 117 North Elm Street, PO Box 1247, Gaylord, MI 49735. Tel: 517-732-3866; Fax: 517-732-6164. (**1989**)

COST: $$$

SAMPLE: Motor Perseveration

"When I tap once, you tap twice. When I tap twice, you tap once."

❏ Mini-Mental State (MMS)

AUTHORS: Marshall F. Folstein, Susan E. Folstein, and Paul R. McHugh

FORMAT: Standardized oral questionnaire.

PURPOSE: This test was developed as a short and simple quantitative measure of cognitive performance. It is intended for clinical use in routine and serial examinations of mental status.

POPULATION: It was designed for use with neuro-geriatric patients, particularly useful for those able to cooperate for short periods only. (Sample consisted of 206 patients in a private psychiatric hospital in New York and 63 normal subjects in a Senior Center and retirement apartment complex.)

SETTING OR POSITION: Not prescribed.

MATERIALS OR TOOLS: Questionnaire, wrist watch, pencil, four sheets of plain blank paper.

METHOD: The questionnaire consists of 11 questions in 5 areas of cognition: orientation, registration (memory), attention and calculation, recall, and language (following oral and written instructions). Each item is scored up to a maximum value; item scores are totalled to a maximum score of 30. The test is not timed and requires 5 to 10 minutes to administer.

INTERPRETATION: The mean score for the normal sample was 27.6, with a range of 24–30. MMS scores identify subjects with cognitive disturbance and quantitatively follow changes in recovery.

RELIABILITY: Test–retest reliability with a 24-hour interval is .887; with two examiners, it is .82. Test–retest reliability for clinically stable patients (elderly depressed and demented) over a 28-day interval is .98.

VALIDITY: MMS scores discriminated among diagnostic categories and distinguished cognitive disorders from the normal group, reflecting presence as well as severity of disability. In patients with improving cognitive status, scores reflect improvement. Concurrent validity was demonstrated in correlations with the Wechsler Adult Intelligence Scale: .776 correlation of MMS with Verbal IQ, .66 of MMS with Performance IQ.

SOURCE: Folstein, M.F., Folstein, S.E., & McHugh, P.R. Minimental state: a practical method for grading the cognitive-state of patients for the clinician. *Journal of Psychiatric Research, 12,* 189–198. (**1975**)

COST: ¢

SAMPLE: Attention and Calculation

Serial 7's [i.e., count by sevens, e.g., 7, 14, 21, etc.]. 1 point for each correct. Stop after 5 answers.

Alternatively, spell "world" backwards.

❒ Mullen Scales of Early Learning: AGS Edition

AUTHOR: Eileen M. Mullen, EdD

FORMAT: Norm-based task performance scales.

PURPOSE: The Mullen Scales are intended as a comprehensive measure of cognitive function for infants and preschool children. Used in a clinical or school setting, they offer a variety of interesting tasks to engage the young child in order to identify strengths and weaknesses and plan intervention.

POPULATION: Children from birth through 68 months (5 years) of age. (The standardization sample consisted of 1,849 children from 2 days to 69 months of age from over 100 sites in 4 geographic regions of the U.S.)

SETTING OR POSITION: Room at a comfortable temperature, with hard surface floor, table, several adult-size chairs, and several colorful toys; an examining table is useful for young infants. Environmental and positioning requirements are described for each scale or item.

MATERIALS OR TOOLS: The kit includes the manual, item administration book, stimulus book, record forms, and a large number of manipulatives and stimulus items; in addition, the examiner needs to provide common items such as cereal, paper, coins, ball, toys, stairs, bench, and a pencil. Computer software is available for scoring and interpretative reports.

METHOD: There are a total of 159 items divided into five Mullen Scales: Gross Motor, Visual Reception, Fine Motor, Receptive Language, and Expressive Language. Before testing, biographical information is recorded and chronological age is computed to indicate starting points for testing. For each item administered, the response is recorded and scored according to directions (e.g., 0 or 1, 1–5 points, etc.). Raw scores may be expressed as T scores, percentile ranks, age equivalents, descriptive categories, and developmental stages. Observations of performance may also be recorded. The scales typically require 15 minutes for 1-year-olds, 30 minutes for 3-year-olds, and 60 minutes for 5-year-olds.

INTERPRETATION: The assessment yields normative scores for each of the 5 scales, which indicate strengths and weaknesses and can be used to plan intervention. The profile of performance across the scales as well as the pattern within each scale helps with planning individualized educational programming. The single composite or summary score represents general intelligence.

RELIABILITY: Item analysis with the Rasch model was used to combine item sets for 5 continuous scales in a single infant–preschool edition. Internal consistency using split-half reliability ranged from .75–.83, with the composite median value of .91. Test–retest reliability with a 1- to 2-week interval ranged from .71–.96. Interrater reliability between paired evaluators ranged from .91 –.99.

VALIDITY: Construct validity is demonstrated by the developmental progression of scores with increasing ages, by intercorrelations of the scales, and by factor analysis supporting the composite score as a measure of general cognitive ability. Concurrent validity is demonstrated by correlations with other measures of development, language, and motor abilities; by prediction to school readiness; and by discriminating between low-birthweight and normal children.

SOURCE: American Guidance Service, Inc., Publishers' Building, Circle Pines, MN 55014. Tel: 800-328-2560; Fax: 612-786-9077. (**1995**)

COST: $$$$

SAMPLE: Gross Motor

Held upright, holds head steady

Materials: none

Position: upright (Up)

Directions: Hold the infant in an upright position against your shoulder, without supporting his/her (see illustration).

Count the number of seconds the infant is able to hold his/her head steady without support.

Scoring: 1 point if the infant holds his/her head steady without support for 12 or more seconds.

❐ Peabody Picture Vocabulary Test-Revised (PPVT)

AUTHORS: Lloyd M. and Leota M. Dunn

FORMAT: Standardized, individually administered screening test.

PURPOSE: The test measures receptive hearing vocabulary for standard American English without requiring verbal or written responses. It provides a simple and quick estimate of one dimension of language comprehension, and is useful in schools, clinics, and vocational and research situations.

POPULATION: Children through adults. Extensive research has been done using samples of people who are disabled and mentally disturbed; research also has been done on using modified administration methods. (PPVT was standardized on ages 2-1/2 to 40 years.)

SETTING OR POSITION: Well-lighted room, undisturbed; two chairs and table, arranged according to manual.

MATERIALS OR TOOLS: Set of test plates, individual test record, pencil.

METHOD: The test consists of a series of 175 plates, graduated in difficulty and bound as an easel. Each plate contains four pictures. The examiner shows each plate and states the corresponding vocabulary word. The subject points to, or otherwise indicates, the picture corresponding to the word. The test begins at the level recommended for the subject being examined and ends following a prescribed pattern of errors, requiring 20 minutes or less to administer. Two equivalent forms, L and M, are available to allow an alternate form in repeated administrations.

INTERPRETATION: The test yields a raw score, which can be converted to age-based norms.

RELIABILITY: Split-half reliability ranged from .67 to .88 (median .80) on Form L and .61 to .86 (median .81) on Form M for ages 2-1/2 through 18. Alternate forms reliability ranged from .73 to .91 (median .82) for raw scores of same age group, and .71 to .89 (median .79) for standard scores. Delayed alternate forms ranged from .52 to .90 (median .78) for raw scores, and .54 to .90 (median .77) for standard scores.

VALIDITY: Content validity is based on dictionary search. Construct validity is based on reported evidence from other intelligence tests of correlations between hearing vocabulary and intelligence. Concurrent validity is demonstrated by high correlations of the revised version with the original PPVT, which correlated with other intelligence and achievement tests.

SOURCE: Published by: American Guidance Service, Inc., Publishers' Building, Circle Pines, MN 55014. Tel: 800-328-2560; Fax: 612-786-9077. [Note: new revision planned 1997] **(1959, revised 1981)**

COST: $

SAMPLE: "I will say a word, and I want you to tell me the number of, or point to, the picture which best tells the meaning of the word."

❏ Prospective Memory Screening (PROMS)

AUTHORS: McKay Moore Sohlberg, PhD, and Catherine A. Mateer, PhD

FORMAT: Performance test, including paper-and-pencil questionnaire.

PURPOSE: PROMS is designed to assess the ability to initiate and carry out planned actions at designated times. The authors suggest that evaluation of prospective memory (remembering to do things at appropriate times) may have greater functional implications than evaluation of retrospective memory or recall (remembering things or events in the past). PROMS offers an effective screening tool that can guide treatment planning.

POPULATION: Not specified. (The sample consisted of 34 normal subjects ages 20 to 59, and 25 brain-injured patients ages 21 to 56 who were participating in inpatient or outpatient rehabilitation and had sustained the injury at least one year before.)

SETTING OR POSITION: Not prescribed, but assumed that subject is seated at a table.

MATERIALS OR TOOLS: PROMS test kit includes manual, Memory Questionnaire, Math Problem Sheet, and stimulus materials. Additional materials are needed: clock or watch with second hand, pencil and paper, penny, envelope, cup, and stamped postcard addressed to examiner.

METHOD: PROMS consists of seven prospective memory tasks requiring the subject to perform a specific task at specified time intervals (1, 2, 10, and 20 minutes, and a 24-hour interval). There may be an overlap of two tasks at a time. Task responses are cued either by time (subject watches the clock) or by associated task (e.g., examiner snaps fingers). Two distractor tasks are provided: a memory questionnaire and a set of math problems to fill out during the time intervals. The math problems can be replaced by an equivalent drawing or writing task for subjects who cannot perform the calculations. Each item is scored one point for each correct response produced at the correct time. The scoresheet allows examiner to note correct response action and time, use of strategies by subject, and performance differences between associate and time cue tasks. Total score ranges from 1 to 7. PROMS requires approximately 1 hour to administer.

INTERPRETATION: Preliminary data from the population sample suggest scoring categories of impaired (1–4), borderline impaired (5), and not impaired (6–7). The Memory Questionnaire may be used by the examiner or trainer for information on the subject's current memory abilities and strategies. The time of the longest task successfully completed is suggested to reflect the limit of the subject's ability. Prospective Memory Training Programs (PROMT) are described to improve prospective memory through intensive training and generalize the skill to functional applications.

RELIABILITY: Pilot data do not offer reliability statistics. The sensitivity of items to the level of impairment varied, indicating tasks of differing levels of difficulty.

VALIDITY: The literature supports the construct of prospective memory as distinct from retrospective memory (test sample exhibited wide variation of scores between PROMS and Randt Memory test of recall), its functional utility, length of prospective memory, and strategies to successfullly complete tasks.

SOURCE: National Rehabilitation Services, 117 North Elm Street, PO Box 1247, Gaylord, MI 49735. Tel: 517-732-3866; Fax: 517-732-6164. (**1989**)

COST: $$$

SAMPLE: Ten minute prospective memory task with time cue.

DIRECTIONS: In exactly ten minutes from right now.....(pause), I would like you to put the penny in the envelope. ...While you are waiting, I would like you to fill out this memory questionnaire.

☐ The Rivermead Behavioural Memory Test (RBMT)

AUTHORS: Barbara Wilson, PhD, Janet Cockburn, and Alan Baddeley

FORMAT: Standardized battery of behavioral and performance skills.

PURPOSE: RBMT is designed to detect and identify memory impairments that occur in everyday activity. By assessing practical rather than experimental application of memory, RBMT can reveal which everyday problems memory-impaired subjects will face, and quantify the frequency or severity of such problems. In addition, it is used to identify areas of treatment and monitor change. It is short and easy to use and interpret.

POPULATION: Norms are available for subjects ages 5 to 11 years (refer to Children's Manual), 11 to 16 years, 16 to 69 years, and 70 to 95 years (refer to Supplement 3, published in 1989). (Original sample consisted of 176 brain-damaged patients at Rivermead Rehabilitation Centre and 118 control subjects. The sample of elderly subjects consisted of 114 people between 70 and 94 years ranging from living at home to community hospital patients. The children's sample consisted of 335 children, ages 5 to 11, from nine schools in Hampshire, England.)

SETTING OR POSITION: A room with table and chair, window, and door is suggested. Bedside or ward administration is not recommended.

MATERIALS OR TOOLS: RBMT kit containing manual, procedural guide and scoring sheet, audiotape (test administration), 1-hour timer, three sets of photographs and line drawings, message envelope, and supplements containing research and normative data; and a pencil. There are separate children's and elderly versions in supplemental manuals; the children's version includes gold stars and several extra pictures and questions.

METHOD: The battery consists of 11 items that must be given in sequence; administration time is less than 30 minutes. The test items involve the following tasks: demonstrating verbal recall, remembering to do a task later in the test, remembering and identifying pictures or drawings, remembering and retelling a story, and retracing a route around the room. In many items, the response is delayed with distractors (other test items in-between). Written directions and scoring procedures are given for each item. The raw score is either the number of items recalled correctly, or how correct or independent the response is (e.g., recalled without prompt=2, with prompt=1, not recalled=0). Four parallel versions allow repeated testing while avoiding the effects of practice. Separate procedures and scoring systems are included in the children's manual.

INTERPRETATION: There are two scoring systems for the RBMT, a Screening Score and a Standardized Profile Score calculated from the subject's Raw Score. The Screening Score ranges from 0–12, and is based on a pass/fail grade for each item. The Standardized Profile Score allocates a score of 2 points (normal), 1 point (borderline), or 0 points (abnormal) for each item. Both scoring systems give cut off points for level of memory function: normal, poor memory, moderately impaired, and severely impaired. The authors offer their own clinically based assessment of the relationship between RBMT scores and everyday performance. Separate interpretation is offered for the elderly in Supplement 3 and for children in the children's manual.

RELIABILITY: Interrater reliability of 1.00 was established by 10 raters, 2 raters each scoring 40 subjects separately but simultaneously. Parallel-form reliability ranged from .67 to .84 on the Screening Score and .83 to .88 on the Standardized Profile Score. Test–retest reliability was established at .78 for the Screening Score and .85 for the Standardized Profile Score; only one item showed significant improvement on second testing.

VALIDITY: RBMT discriminated between brain-damaged and control subjects who received substantially higher scores. RBMT scores demonstrated significant correlations with standard test scores from other memory tests, therapists' daily memory checklists, and subjective ratings by patients and relatives (as extrapolated from correlations with memory test scores). The validity study examines the effects of intelligence, location of lesion, dysphasia, and perceptual problems on RBMT performance and how to adjust testing accordingly. Supplement 3 addresses these issues separately for elderly subjects. Interestingly, there was little evidence overall of patterns or clusters of specific memory deficits.

SOURCE: Published by Thames Valley Test Company, Suffolk, England. Distributed in North America by: National Rehabilitation Services, 117 North Elm, PO Box 1247, Gaylord, MI 49735. Tel: 517-732-3866; Fax: 517-732-6164. (**1991**)

COST: $$$

SAMPLE: Belonging

Say: 'What I am going to do now is to put something of yours away, and see if you can remember to ask me for it when I say we have finished this test. I also want you to remember where I put it. ...'

❐ Routine Task Inventory (RTI-2)

AUTHOR: Claudia Kay Allen, MA, OTR, FAOTA

FORMAT: Performance rating scale based on observation, self-report, and/or structured interview.

PURPOSE: The RTI was developed as a measure of impairment as it relates to the performance of activities of daily living. This method of describing performance utilizes the ratings from Allen's Theory of Cognitive Levels.

POPULATION: Adults who may have cognitive impairments; the RTI was originally developed for use in psychiatric hospitals. (Information on the research sample is not included in the text.)

SETTING OR POSITION: Customary setting for observing daily activity; not prescribed for report or interview format.

MATERIALS OR TOOLS: Scoresheet, questionnaire, and a pencil.

METHOD: RTI-2 consists of four behavior (cognitive) disabilities, each comprising eight activities that are likely to be important to most people. The four disabilities are: self-awareness (consisting of self-care activities), situational awareness (home and community activities), occupational role disability (e.g., planning, organizing, exerting effort), and social role disability (meeting social expectations when interacting with others). Each item is described by general activity analysis. Three methods may be used to administer the RTI-2: caregiver report (a fast, reliable indication of the pattern of subject's performance), self-report by the subject (depending on cognitive level), and observation of performance. A questionnaire is provided to describe each activity and manner of performance. Criteria are given for rating each item from 1–6 at each cognitive level that applies.

INTERPRETATION: The ratings offer a way of describing behavior according to the level of cognitive ability. When more than one rating method is used, scores can be compared to demonstrate discrepancies between self-report (that is, subject's awareness) and observer's or caregiver's report.

RELIABILITY: Studies on the original RTI established significant interrater reliability of .98) and test–retest reliability of .91 (.99 in a second study). Internal consistency was .94, reflecting task equivalence among activities.

VALIDITY: Correlation between RTI and Allen Cognitive Level was .56, and .61 between RTI and Mini-Mental State in a population with senile dementia.

SOURCE: Published in: Allen, C.K., Earhart, C.A., & Blue, T. *Occupational therapy treatment goals for the physically and cognitively disabled* (pp. 54–68). Bethesda, MD: American Occupational Therapy Association. **(1992)**

COST: $

SAMPLE: Contributing to Family Activities

(level) 3. Efforts to participate in family activities are disruptive or demand constant attention from at least one other person at all times.
4. Participates in a restricted range of family activities.
5. Participates in full range of family activities.
May not contribute new ideas for future planning and decision making, or
May not place other members' interests ahead of own interest, or engage in give and take gracefully.

❑ Severe Impairment Battery (SIB)

AUTHORS: J. Saxton, K. L. McGonigle, A. A. Swihart, and F. Boller

FORMAT: Performance test and rating scale.

PURPOSE: SIB was developed to assess the low end of the range of cognitive function in patients who are too impaired to complete standard neuropsychological tests. The assessment demonstrates performance on low-level tasks and follows patterns of deterioration over time.

POPULATION: Severely demented older adults. (Sample consisted of 70 patients, ages 51–91, fom the University of Pittsburgh Alzheimer's Disease Research Center who met criteria for probable or possible AD.)

SETTING OR POSITION: Quiet room with subject seated comfortably at a desk or table, facing examiner who carefully maintains eye contact.

MATERIALS OR TOOLS: Test pack includes manual, questionnaire, summary chart, blocks, utensils, board; and a pencil. Common distractor items are provided by the examiner.

METHOD: This 20-minute test is composed of very simple one-step commands that are presented in conjunction with gestural cues. After rapport is established, items are presented in a smoothly flowing interview-like sequence designed to elicit natural or automatic responses. The items are organized in six subscales: attention, orientation, language, memory, visuospatial ability, and construction. Also included are brief evaluations of praxis, ability to respond appropriately to being called by name, and an assessment of social interaction skills. Most items are scored on a 3-point scale: 2=correct, 1=partially correct (or gesture to demonstrate correct answer), and 0=incorrect. Scores are totalled for a range of 0–100.

INTERPRETATION: The severity of impairment is graded as reflected by the score; a total score of less than 63 indicates very severe impairment. Scores on individual subscales indicate patterns of impairment that may be compared over time and with the course of neuropsychological decline.

RELIABILITY: Interrater reliability with two raters simultaneously scoring 24 subjects was .99 for the total score, with a range of .89–1.0 on the subscales. Test–retest reliability was .90 for total score, with an interval of 30 days or less; widely varying subscale correlations are possibly due to day-to-day changes in the subjects.

VALIDITY: Correlations of SIB scores with the Mini-Mental State Examination and the Mattis Dementia Rating Scale were .76 and .88 respectively, and .47 and .85 in the very severely demented population (which may reflect limitations of the MMSE scoring). Validation studies on an earlier version resulted in minor changes to eliminate redundant items; further studies are in progress. Similar reliability and validity correlations resulted from a French version administered in a suburb of Paris; in addition, SIB differentiated among severity groups classified by MMSE scores.

SOURCE: Published by Thames Valley Test Company, Suffolk, England. Distributed in North America by: National Rehabilitation Services, 117 North Elm, Street PO Box 1247, Gaylord, MI 49735. Tel: 517-732-3866. Fax: 517-732-6164. (**1993**)

COST: $$$

SAMPLE: Language

Show round block say "What shape is this?"	2 points: spontaneously correct
If no response prompt: say "Is this a triangle or a square?"	1 point: if correct after prompt, or "pyramid"

❑ Short Portable Mental Status Questionnaire (SPMSQ)

AUTHOR: Eric Pfeiffer, MD

FORMAT: Oral questionnaire.

PURPOSE: This mental status examination is intended to provide a brief, simple, reliable instrument to detect the presence and degree of intellectual impairment. It can be helpful in diagnosing or planning treatment for patients with organic brain deficit who cannot cooperate with complex testing.

POPULATION: Elderly patients. (Sample consisted of 997 elderly people in North Carolina living in the community, plus 141 referred for clinic evaluation, and 102 living in institutions.)

SETTING OR POSITION: Not prescribed.

MATERIALS OR TOOLS: Test sheet, instructions, and pencil.

METHOD: SPMSQ consists of 10 questions testing diverse aspects of intellectual functioning, including short-term and remote memory, orientation to surroundings, information about current events, and serial mathematical tasks. Each question is asked of the subject, and answers are recorded. Criteria are given for scoring correct responses. The score is based on the total number of errors and ranges from 0–10. The level of education and race of the subject is recorded on the test sheet.

INTERPRETATION: The scores, adjusted for subjects' race and education, yield four levels, ranging from intact intellectual functioning to severe intellectual impairment. Capacity for self-care is derived from this classification, ranging from intellectually capable of self-care to probable diagnosis of organic brain syndrome and requiring continuous supervision of activities.

RELIABILITY: Test–retest correlations of .82 and .83 were obtained for two groups of subjects aged 65 or over, with a four-week test interval. The author described these correlations as remarkably stable.

VALIDITY: Face validity is apparent from the difference in distribution-of-error scores between the community sample and the institutional sample who received poorer scores. Comparing SPMSQ scores with clinical diagnosis, there was .92 agreement on those judged impaired by each method, .82 agreement on no or mild impairment, and .88 agreement between moderate to severe impairment and a diagnosis of organic brain syndrome.

SOURCE: Pfeiffer, E. A short portable mental status questionnaire for the assessment of organic brain deficit in elderly patients. *Journal of the American Geriatrics Society, 23*(10), 433–441. (1975)

COST: ¢

SAMPLE: What is your telephone number?

◻ Test of Everyday Attention (TEA)

AUTHORS: Ian H. Robertson, Tony Ward, Valerie Ridgeway, and Ian Nimmo-Smith

FORMAT: Battery of visual- and auditory-based performance tasks.

PURPOSE: The TEA is designed to test attention systems that are believed to be independent in the brain, serving different functions in everyday behavior. Using familiar materials and tasks, it should be useful in identifying attention-related problems and predicting recovery of function over time.

POPULATION: Adults. (Sample consisted of 154 normal subjects, ages 18 to 80 divided into four age bands and two educational levels, and 80 patients two months postunilateral cerebrovascular accident [CVA].)

SETTING OR POSITION: A quiet, well-lit location with a flat surface for the test materials. Examiner should sit at a right angle to the subject.

MATERIALS OR TOOLS: The test kit includes the manual, spiral-bound test materials book, scoresheets, plastic-coated maps and telephone directory pages, and colored pens. In addition, a stopwatch and cassette recorder are needed.

METHOD: There are eight subtests of the TEA that are sensitive to four types of attention identified: selective attention, sustained attention, attentional switching, and divided (auditory–verbal) attention. The subtests involve various visual and auditory tasks such as searching for symbols in a telephone book or map and listening for digits in lottery numbers. Scoring instructions differ with each subtest and are based on time and/or accuracy. There are three parallel versions of the TEA which allow for repeated testing. Administration takes from 45 minutes to 1 hour.

INTERPRETATION: Raw scores are converted to scaled scores (adjusted scores that can be compared with each other) and percentiles to compare with the sample. Scaled scores falling in the shaded area of the scoresheet (7% or below) indicate probable abnormality. The authors offer brief guides to interpretation for each subtest as well as general guidelines regarding functional implications of the four attention factors.

RELIABILITY: Test–retest reliability for normal and post-CVA subjects, with a 1-week interval, on subtest scores of two parallel versions of the test, ranged from .59–.90 for normal subjects and .77–.90 for CVA patients with one exception of a task that may have demonstrated learning.

VALIDITY: The manual summarizes correlations between two subtests and three other functional assessments in testing CVA patients. Subtest scores were found to discriminate between control subjects and patients with CVA or closed head injury. Factor analysis identified the degree to which the four attentional factors were measured in every subtest. Interfering factors to testing, such as impaired hearing or visual acuity, are accommodated.

SOURCE: Published by Thames Valley Test Company, Suffolk, England. Distributed in North America by: National Rehabilitation Services, 117 North Elm Street, PO Box 1247, Gaylord, MI 49735. Tel: 517-732-3866; Fax: 517-732-6164. **(1994)**

COST: $$$

SAMPLE: Map Search

The symbol here (show symbol from cuebook) shows where restaurants can be found in the Philadelphia area. …What I would like you to do is to look at the map for two minutes and circle as many symbols as you can. …

❑ Test of Orientation for Rehabilitation Patients (TORP)

AUTHORS: Jean Dietz, PhD, OTR/L, FAOTA, Clara Beeman, MOT, OTR/L, and Deborah Thorn, MS, OTR/L

FORMAT: Standard verbal question-and-answer test.

PURPOSE: This thorough, quantitative measure of orientation is designed to determine the existence and extent of disorientation, establish a baseline level of performance, plan intervention, monitor patient progress, and assess the effectiveness of rehabilitative treatment.

POPULATION: Adults and adolescents who have been in treatment for a minimum of 1 week in inpatient rehabilitation settings, including those with head trauma, cerebrovascular accident (CVA), seizure disorder, brain tumor, or any other neurological condition resulting in confusion and disorientation. It is contraindicated for those with significant aphasia.

SETTING OR POSITION: Quiet, distraction-free room with no cues that might help with test questions (e.g., clock, wristwatch). If the subject is seated at a table, the table should be bare. The test is administered individually, ideally in one session, but must be completed in the same day.

MATERIALS OR TOOLS: Test manual, test booklet (correct answers unique to the subject are recorded before testing), and pencil.

METHOD: The TORP consists of 46 items sampling five domains of orientation: orientation to person and personal situation, place, time, schedule, and temporal continuity. Each test item is an open-ended verbal question, with an auditory recognition (i.e., multiple choice) alternate in case the subject fails to answer correctly. Only verbal responses are required, but the test can be adapted for use by nonverbal patients with communication aids. Test instructions, response procedures for the examiner, and scoring criteria are given. Each item is scored SC (Spontaneous Correct), RC (Recognition Correct), or I (Incorrect). The entire test is timed. The manual includes a self-study module to train examiners in test administration and scoring.

INTERPRETATION: TORP Score Sheet yields raw scores and percentage scores for each domain from which total scores are calculated. Scores can be graphed on the daily or weekly graph of total test scores for comparison. To assist in interpreting total test and domain corrected scores, a table is offered with low and high scores and percentile scores for 35 rehabilitation patients without brain injuries.

RELIABILITY: Reliability studies were conducted with subjects with and without brain injuries and at least 14 years of age. Interrater reliability subscores ranged from .89 to 1.00 (test total .98) for the group without injury, and .94 to .99 (test total .99) for the group with brain injury. Test–retest reliability of total scores with a 3-to-5-day interval were .85 for the group without brain injury and .95 for the group with brain injury.

VALIDITY: A review of the literature and consultation with experts yielded test items which were reviewed by an interdisciplinary group of experts in the field of brain injury; content experts judged item–objective congruence, categorizing 46 test items in the domains they best measured. Construct validity was demonstrated by higher TORP scores of rehabilitation patients with brain injuries as compared to those without brain injuries.

SOURCE: Therapy Skill Builders, a division of Psychological Corporation, 555 Academic Court, San Antonio, Texas 78204-2498. Tel: 800-228-0752; Fax: 800-232-1223. **(1993)**

COST: $$

SAMPLE: What day of the week comes after Thursday? _____

Recognition: Is the day of the week that comes after Thursday...?

                    Saturday   Monday   Wednesday or   Friday

Accept: Friday

Psychological

Assessments

❐ Internal/External Scale

AUTHOR: J. B. Rotter

FORMAT: Forced-choice questionnaire.

PURPOSE: The test provides a unidimensional measure of the individual's belief in internal versus external control over the consequences of personal action, that is, whether individuals control their own behavior (internal control) or are influenced by forces outside of their own control (external control).

POPULATION: Older adolescents and adults. The test requires sufficient reading ability to render it unsuitable below the junior high school level. (Research is based on college student samples; over 4,000 subjects contributed to the normative data.)

SETTING OR POSITION: Not prescribed, but test results are sensitive to or influenced by the setting.

MATERIALS OR TOOLS: Questionnaire and pencil.

METHOD: The test consists of 23 question-pairs plus six filler questions. In each item, the respondent chooses one of two alternative statements. The statements represent polar views of internal and external control and the respondent's choice reflects personal belief. The questionnaire is scored according to a key and yields a single score. Administration time is approximately 15 minutes.

INTERPRETATION: Score indicates degree of externality, ranging from 0 (most internal) to 23 (most external). Relative internality is desirable, and an external locus of control orientation is considered an obstacle toward getting along in society. Intervention may be indicated for personal change as well as for change in the immediate environment (Robinson & Shaver, 1973). Rotter's discussion guides interpretation of the score.

RELIABILITY: Internal consistency is .70; test–retest coefficients were .72 with a 1-month interval and .55 with a 2-month interval. The instrument is sensitive to the circumstances of the administration.

VALIDITY: A wide range of studies generally support discriminant, concurrent, and construct validity. Factor analysis yielded one general primary factor.

SOURCES: Rotter, J. B. (1966). Generalized expectancies for internal versus external control of reinforcement. *Psychological Monographs*, *80*, 1–28.

Also found in: Robinson, J., & Shaver, P. (1973). *Measures of social psychological attitudes* (pp. 227-231). Ann Arbor, MI: Institute of Social Research.

COST: ¢

SAMPLE: a. There are certain people who are just no good.

           b. There is some good in everybody.

❏ Locus of Control for Children

AUTHORS: Stephen Nowicki and Bonnie R. Strickland

FORMAT: Questionnaire.

PURPOSE: The scale, a parallel to Rotter's Internal–External Scale, is designed to measure the same expectations for control in school-age children. As a measure of internal versus external orientation, it indicates whether children feel their personal actions are within or outside of their own control.

POPULATION: School-age children, grades 1–12, capable of reading and responding. The scale has been modified for use with college and adult populations. (Sample consisted of 1,017 children, grades 3 through 12, in four different communities.)

SETTING OR POSITION: Not prescribed.

MATERIALS OR TOOLS: Questionnaire, pencil.

METHOD: The scale is a 40-item self-report task. Two 20-item versions were developed for grades 1 through 6 and grades 7 through 12. Children are asked to indicate agreement or disagreement (yes/no) with statements concerning personal control over outcomes. The scale yields a single score.

INTERPRETATION: Score indicates degree of externality, ranging from 0 (most internal) to 20 (most external) in the shorter version. Relative internality is desirable (see Internal/External Scale).

RELIABILITY: Internal consistency via split-half reliability ranges from .63 (grades 3 to 5) to .81 (grade 12); test–retest reliability with a 6-week interval ranges from .63 (grade 3) to .71 (grade 10).

VALIDITY: Some concurrent and construct validity is evident in varying correlations with other internal/ external tests and achievement scores.

SOURCES: Nowicki, S., & Strickland, B.R. A locus of control scale for children. *Journal of Consulting & Clinical Psychology, 40,* 148–154. **(1973)**

Also found in Robinson, J., & Shaver, P. (1973). *Measures of social psychological attitudes* (pp. 206–211). Ann Arbor, MI: Institute of Social Research.

COST: ¢

SAMPLE: Are you often blamed for things that just aren't your fault?

    (Yes/No)

Do you think that cheering more than luck helps a team to win?

    (Yes/No)

❏ Personal Value Scales

AUTHOR: W. Scott

FORMAT: Rating scale.

PURPOSE: The scales were developed to measure personal values by college students. With the exception of family or work-related values, it otherwise offers a comprehensive picture.

POPULATION: College students (could be modified for adults). Sample consisted of over 900 students from University of Colorado fraternities and sororities.)

SETTING OR POSITION: Not prescribed.

MATERIALS OR TOOLS: Questionnaire, pencil.

METHOD: Twelve categories of values are examined, each containing four to six items: short form is a 1/2-hour 60-item test, long form is a 1-hour (or more) 240-item test. The categories are: intellectualism, kindness, social skills, loyalty, academic achievement, physical development, status, honesty, religiousness, self-control, creativity, and independence. Items are rated from Always Admire (usually 1 point)–Depends on Situation–Always Dislike (both 0 points).

INTERPRETATION: Each value scale yields a summed score, which indicates the relative importance of the category to the individual. The values generally reflect judgments of right/wrong or good/bad in interpersonal relations (Robinson & Shaver, 1973).

RELIABILITY: Long form has higher consistency (ranges .80–.89 versus .55–.78 on short form); test–retest is variable for short form (.58–.77). Correlations between the two forms range from .62–.85.

VALIDITY: Concurrent validity is reported high, based on student ratings on the items according to related qualities (e.g., rightness and wrongness). Scores were found to discriminate among groups with expected qualities (e.g., art majors and creativity).

SOURCE: Originally published in: Scott, W. *Values and organizations: A study of fraternities and sororities.* Chicago: RandMcNally. (Out of print but available in over 400 U.S. libraries.) **(1965)**

Robinson, J., & Shaver, P. (1973). *Measures of social psychological attitudes.* Ann Arbor, MI: Institute for Social Research.

COST: ¢

SAMPLE:	Always admire	Depends on situation	Always dislike	
[check one]				Being popular with everyone

❑ Philadelphia Geriatric Center Morale Scale

AUTHOR: M. Powell Lawton, PhD

FORMAT: Interview (oral recommended over written).

PURPOSE: This scale was designed to operationalize morale as multidimensional, rather than unidimensional, and provide a simple and understandable tool for measuring it among the very old.

POPULATION: Elderly, over 70 years of age; simplicity of wording and response forms are especially appropriate for very old and less competent individuals. (Mean scores are based on a sample of 928 respondents.)

SETTING OR POSITION: Not prescribed.

MATERIALS OR TOOLS: Questionnaire, User's Guide, and a pencil.

METHOD: The original 22-item scale defined 6 dimensions of morale; a revised 17-item scale identifies 3 dimensions resulting from factor analysis. They are: agitation, attitude toward own aging, and lonely dissatisfaction. The respondent replies "yes" or "no" to most questions, one point given to each high morale response.

INTERPRETATION: A total morale score is obtained, as well as scores for the three factors.

RELIABILITY: Split-half reliability is .79, internal consistency is .81, and test–retest reliability ranges from .75-.91. Revised scale: three factors have high degree of internal consistency (.85, .81, .85).

VALIDITY: Moderately concurrent with life satisfaction scores (.57, .76, .79) and judge's ratings (.47); morale also correlated with numerous factors in activities (e.g., social interaction, employment, mobility).

SOURCES: Obtain from author at: Philadelphia Geriatric Center, 5301 Old York Road, Philadelphia, PA 19141.

Tel: 215-456-2004, extension 2979.

Lawton, M.P. (1975). The Philadelphia Geriatric Center Morale Scale. *Journal of Gerontology, 30*, 85–89.

Lawton, M.P. (1972). The dimensions in morale. In D. Kent, R. Kastenbaum, & S. Sherwood (Eds.), *Research, planning, and action for the elderly*. New York: Behavioral Publications.

COST: ¢

SAMPLE: "Sometimes I worry so much that I can't sleep."

"As you get older, you are less useful."

❏ Piers-Harris Childrens Self-Concept Scale

AUTHORS: Ellen V. Piers, PhD and Dale B. Harris, PhD

FORMAT: Standardized self-report questionnaire.

PURPOSE: This test is designed to measure self-concept, that is, conscious self-perceptions (self-esteem, self-regard), in children and adolescents. It can be used in routine screening in high-risk settings, as an aid to individual assessment for counseling, and as a research tool (e.g., to study treatment outcome).

POPULATION: Children and adolescents, ages 8 to 18; contraindicated for those unable or unwilling to cooperate with the scales. Studies are summarized describing specialized use with children of various ethnic and disability groups. (Normative sample is based on 1,183 public school pupils from a small town in Pennsylvania in the early 1960s. Additional norms are available from a variety of populations, totalling 3,692 normal school children.)

SETTING OR POSITION: Quiet, well-lit room, free of distractions, with a hard writing surface and a comfortable chair.

MATERIALS: Manual, 4-page test booklet, and a soft-leaded pencil with eraser.

METHOD: The test is an 80-item self-report questionnaire consisting of statements reflecting how children feel about themselves, to which the subject responds "yes" or "no." The scale yields a total raw score, percentile score, overall stanine score, and conversion to normalized T-scores. Six cluster scores are provided to aid interpretation: Behavior, Intellectual and School Status, Physical Appearance and Attributes, Anxiety, Popularity, and Happiness and Satisfaction. It can be administered individually or in groups. Administration and scoring require fewer than 30 minutes.

INTERPRETATION: Total score is compared to the norms: High score suggests positive self-concept, low suggests negative. Relative strengths and weaknesses of the individual can be determined from the cluster scores. Individual item scores may illuminate the individual's results. The authors caution that ultimate responsibility for use and interpretation should remain with those trained in psychological testing, and that it should not be used in isolation of other assessment methods.

RELIABILITY: Test–retest reliability ranges from .42 (with 8-month interval) to .96 (3- to 4-week interval), with median of .73. Additional studies with various population samples are summarized. Internal consistency for total scores range from .88 to .93.

VALIDITY: Content validity is based on selection of qualities that children like or dislike about themselves according to reported studies. Concurrent validity studies compare the instrument with other self-concept measures as well as other behavioral and personality measures. Criterion-related studies indicate that the Piers-Harris scores discriminate among groups. Factor analyses have supported underlying dimensions of self-concept as established in the test. Construct validity studies support the construct of self-concept.

SOURCE: Published by: Western Psychological Services, 12031 Wilshire Boulevard, Los Angeles, CA 90025-1251. Tel: 800-648-8857; Fax: 310-478-7838. (**1969, revised 1984**)

COST: $$

SAMPLE: "I am well behaved in school."

"I get nervous when the teacher calls on me."

❒ Self-Esteem Scale

AUTHOR: M. Rosenberg

FORMAT: Unidimensional self-rating scale.

PURPOSE: The scale provides a quick and simple method of measuring the degree of positive and negative attitudes toward one's abilities and accomplishments.

POPULATION: Developed for use with adolescents, also used in studies of the elderly. Thus, it appears appropriate to a wide age range. (Original sample consisted of 5,024 11th and 12th graders from 10 randomly selected New York schools.)

SETTING OR POSITION: Not prescribed.

MATERIALS OR TOOLS: Written scale and pencil.

METHOD: The scale consists of 10 simple statements describing oneself and is completed in 5 minutes. The subject rates each item along a 4-point continuum ranging from "strongly disagree" to "strongly agree."

INTERPRETATION: The scoring guide yields a ranking of high, medium, or low self-esteem. (Some investigators simply summed the responses.)

RELIABILITY: Reproductibility and scalability coefficients (as used with Guttman Scales such as this) are respectively .92 and .72. Test–retest over a 2-week interval was .85.

VALIDITY: Construct and possibly predictive validity is based on correlations of self-esteem to other personality traits and levels of activity (e.g., less shyness, more assertive, more extracurricular activities). Additional correlations are made with ratings by peers and professionals. Correlations are also found with several similar measures and with clinical assessment.

SOURCES: Rosenberg, M. *Society and the adolescent self-image.* Princeton, NJ: Princeton University Press. (**1965**)

Robinson, J., & Shaver, P. (1973). *Measures of social psychological attitudes* (pp. 81–83). Ann Arbor, MI: Institute of Social Research.

COST: ¢

SAMPLE: I wish I could have more respect for myself. [Rate from "strongly agree" to "strongly disagree."]

□ SHORT-CARE (as derived from CARE, Comprehensive Assessment and Referral Evaluation)

AUTHORS: Barry Gurland, MD, Robert R. Golden, PhD, Jeanne A. Teresi, EdD, and Judith Challop, PhD

FORMAT: Rating scale based on semi-structured interview.

PURPOSE: CARE and SHORT-CARE systematically assess the medical, psychiatric, and social functions and dysfunctions of elderly adults. SHORT-CARE is shorter and more selective, recommended to occupational therapists for assessing depression, dementia, and disability.

POPULATION: Community-based elderly population, aged 65 and over. (CARE was developed from a cross-national U.S./U.K. sample in New York and London of 866 elderly people living in the community and 175 psychogeriatric and geriatric medical patients; 1,131 people in the community and 30 health center patients participated in the CARE pilot study; SHORT-CARE used data from this sample as well as from a national hypertension study in the U.S.)

SETTING OR POSITION: Unspecified community or home setting; private area is needed for the interview.

MATERIALS OR TOOLS: Instruction manual, interview packet, scoresheet, and pencil.

METHOD: The original CARE contains 1,500 items and requires 1 1/2 hours to administer. SHORT-CARE is reduced to 143 items requiring over 30 minutes to administer. In part one, the interviewer asks specified true/false questions regarding the subject's symptoms during the previous month. Responses are judged and recorded according to defined ratings. In part two, additional items provide operational diagnoses and screen out cases without dementia and/or depression. Training is required for obtaining and administering SHORT-CARE.

INTERPRETATION: Cut-off scores indicate the individual is at risk for depression, dementia, or disability (i.e., dependence). Six heterogeneous indicator scales are derived from scores in part one, each denoting a health or social problem: depression/ demoralization, organic brain syndrome (dementia), subjective memory impairment, sleep disorders, somatic symptoms, and activity limitation (disabilty). The operational diagnoses derived from part two (pervasive depression, pervasive dementia, and personal time dependency [disability]) identify a need for clinical investigation or intervention.

RELIABILITY: The SHORT-CARE demonstrates satisfactory interrater reliability for the three impairments, depression, dementia, and disability (.94, .76, .91 respectively); internal consistency for the impairments is .75, .64, .81 and for operational diagnoses is .82, .88, .78. (A test of interrater reliability using videotaped interview is required of all examiners.)

VALIDITY: The validity of SHORT-CARE is based in part on its psychometric association with CARE, one of the most widely tested multidimensional instruments. The homogeneous scales are found to measure unique constructs separately. Diagnostic scales cut across homogeneous scales and prove superior in concurrent and predictive validity. SHORT-CARE has been demonstrated to be a valid screening tool for depression and dementia.

SOURCES: For training and instrument, contact: John Toner, PhD or Patricia A. Miller, MED, OTR, FAOTA, Center for Geriatrics and Gerontology, Columbia University, 100 Haven Avenue—Suite 3-30F, New York, NY 10032. Tel: 212-781-0600.

Golden, R., Teresi, J., & Gurland, B. (1984). Development of Indicator Scales for the Comprehensive Assessment and Referral Evaluation (CARE) Interview Schedule. *Journal of Gerontology, 39*(2), 138–146.

Gurland, B., Golden, R., Teresi, J., & Challop, J. (1984). The SHORT-CARE: An efficient instrument for the assessment of depression, dementia and disability. *Journal of Gerontology, 39*(2), 166–169.

Gurland, B.J., & Wilder, D.E. (1984). The CARE Interview revisited: Development of an efficient, systematic clinical assessment. *Journal of Gerontology, 39*(2), 129–137.

COST: $$$, includes training and materials.

SAMPLE: What kind of things do you worry about?...Your health?...Money?...

Have you been sad or depressed during the past month?

❏ Stanford Preschool Internal-External Scale (SPIES)

AUTHORS: W. Mischel, R. Zeiss, and A. Zeiss

FORMAT: Forced-choice scale administered orally.

PURPOSE: This scale, designed specifically for pre-school-age children, measures internal and external orientation with respect to both positive and negative outcomes of behavior. Three types of situations are addressed: parent–child and peer interactions and control over objects.

POPULATION: Preschool-age children; inappropriate for children with significant communication or cognitive deficits. (Normative sample ranged from 3 years, 2 months to 5 years, 8 months; however, reliability is diminished under age 4.)

SETTING OR POSITION: A room with table, two chairs, and several toys for initial play period.

MATERIALS OR TOOLS: Scale for examiner.

METHOD: The scale consists of two subscales, one of items relating positive, successful, and happy outcomes and one relating unhappy and failing outcomes. Practice questions are posed to accustom the child to the procedure. Then 14 forced-choice items are administered orally, repeating each once for the child to make a choice.

INTERPRETATION: Two scores are obtained: one for control over positive outcomes and one for control over negative outcomes. (See Internal/External Scale for comments.)

RELIABILITY: Test–retest reliability over 4 months was .43 for the positive scale and .64 for the negative scale: adequate for research, but inadequate for clinical use unless corroborated, according to the authors.

VALIDITY: Studies support concurrent validity; positive and negative subscales demonstrated correlations independently, showing that the scale measures two sets of beliefs.

SOURCE: Mischel, W., Zeiss, R., & Zeiss, A. Internal-external control and persistence: Validation and implications of the Stanford Preschool Internal-External Scale. *Journal of Personality and Social Psychology, 29,* 265–278. **(1974)**

COST: ¢

SAMPLE: When you are happy, are you happy:

> a. because you did something fun, or
>
> b. because somebody was nice to you?

❑ Tennessee Self-Concept Scale—Revised (TSCS)

AUTHORS: Gale H. Roid, PhD and William H. Fitts, PhD

FORMAT: Standardized self-administered rating scale.

PURPOSE: The TSCS was developed to provide a simple, widely applicable, and multidimensional assessment of self-concept. It can be used in counseling, clinical evaluation and diagnosis, research, personnel selection, and more.

POPULATION: Adolescents and adults aged 12 or older who can read at approximately a fourth-grade level or higher, ranging from normal through severe psychologically maladjusted individuals. (Original sample consisted of 626 12- to 68-year-olds representing a cross-section of U.S. residents. New norms for the revised version were developed for adolescents based on numerous research studies.)

SETTING OR POSITION: Not prescribed.

MATERIALS OR TOOLS: Manual, test booklet, appropriate answer-profile form, hand-scoring key if needed, no. 2 pencil.

METHOD: The TSCS consists of 100 self-descriptive statements, self-administered individually or in groups in 10 to 20 minutes. The subject is instructed to rate the degree to which each item describes himself or herself using a scale from 1 (Completely False) to 5 (Completely True). Profile validity (i.e. candidness) is checked by the Self-Criticism score (degree to which subject is willing to admit to common frailties) and Distribution score (indicating noncommittal or guarded answers). Additional validity scales are present in the Clinical and Research format. Scoring can be done in any of three formats: computer-scorable (from WPS), hand-scorable Counseling Form (requiring 6–7 minutes), and hand-scorable Clinical and Research Form (30 minutes).

INTERPRETATION: The Counseling scoring format yields 14 scores most relevent to normal functioning subjects, including Total Score reflecting overall level of self-esteem. Clinical and Research format offers 20 scores used primarily for technical research and test development, including several clinical scales for dysfunctional or serious clinical cases. The computer scoring provides detailed interpretation, a group summary if desired, and a color profile of scores in relation to four normative groups: Well-Integrated, Normal, Depressed, and Acting Out. Each TSCS profile can be converted to percentiles and compared with the normative sample.

RELIABILITY: Numerous reliability studies are summarized indicating split-half reliability (.91) and internal consistency (Total Score .92, Self-Criticism .66; subsets achieved above .80 in three samples; inter-item correlations .79; and more). Test–retest reliability over a 2-week interval ranged from .60 to .92, and .88 for Total Score on a shortened version.

VALIDITY: Content validity is based on literature review, items derived from other self-concept measures, and item classification agreement by seven clinical psychologists. Items that differentiated one group from all others were used to compose a specific scale for that group. Evidence of the stability and of the construct validity of the TSCS is discussed, including correlations with other measures of self-concept, other personality measures, and life experiences. Factor analysis yielded evidence of the multidimensionality of the items and scales of the TSCS. Criterion-related studies indicate that test scores discriminate among groups (e.g., psychiatric patients, delinquents, recipients of intervention).

SOURCE: Published by: Western Psychological Services, 12031 Wilshire Boulevard, Los Angeles, CA 90025-1251. **(1988)**

Tel: 800-648-8857; Fax: 310-478-7838.

COST: $$

SAMPLE:

	Completely False	Mostly False	Partly False and Partly True	Mostly True	Completely True

I am satisfied with my family relationships.

I am just as nice as I should be.

❑ Volitional Questionnaire (2nd Edition)

AUTHOR: Carmen Gloria de las Heras, MS, OTR

FORMAT: Rating scale based on observation of behavior and interview.

PURPOSE: Based on the Model of Human Occupation (MOHO), this assessment of volition (including goals, interests, values) is designed for clients who cannot adequately express these ideas verbally. This instrument provides a format for communicating volition through actions and for identifying the optimal conditions and supports needed for this expression.

POPULATION: Individuals with cognitive or verbal limitations; initially developed for mentally retarded and chronic psychiatric clients.

SETTING OR POSITION: The author suggests environments appropriate for the assessment, with general recommendations of available materials and activities, structure, social support, and number of participants. There is great latitude for individualizing the setting according to the needs of the subject.

MATERIALS OR TOOLS: Instructions, questionnaire, nursing staff questionnaire, pencil; in addition, all common materials needed for supplying the environment for activity.

METHOD: The questionnaire contains 14 statements that express components of the three areas of volition: intrinsic motivation, personal causation, and interests/values. These are assessed through observation of performance in up to five activity sessions related to work, daily living, and/or leisure environments. The environment for the activity is prepared in advance, and adapted, if necessary, to the subject's needs. The subject is invited to explore alternative activities and select one to perform, during which the therapist introduces novelty or increasing demands. Afterwards, the therapist and subject discuss feelings related to the activity and environment. Following each observation, the therapist rates each component on a 4-point scale in terms of spontaneity and amount of support, structure, or stimulation needed, and then adds comments and writes a conclusion. Ideally the observations are made in small groups, although they may be done individually. The Nursing Questionnaire serves as a complementary self-care assessment.

INTERPRETATION: The results indicate when and under what conditions the subject demonstrates useful and appropriate volition, and what kind of environment or support facilitates spontaneous expression of interests, values, motivation, and personal causation.

RELIABILITY: Kielhofner (1995) summarizes the unpublished work of the author to conclude that the questionnaire demonstrates reasonable stability and adequate interrater reliability, and supporting the belief that changing environments influence volition.

VALIDITY: Content validity was established through review of the literature and by a panel of MOHO experts, who also found preliminary evidence that the instrument reflected the model constructs. Rasch analysis was used to confirm that the items demonstrate a single construct of volition. Revisions resulting from a study on discriminant validity led to increased ability to discriminate among varying levels of volitional ability; some items may be too easy for less impaired subjects.

SOURCES: Distributed by: Model of Human Occupation Clearinghouse, University of Illinois at Chicago, Department of Occupational Therapy (M/C 811), College of Associated Health Professions, 1919 West Taylor Street, Chicago, IL 60612-7250. Tel: 312-996-6901; Fax: 312-413-0256. (**1988, revised 1994**)

Kielhofner, G. (1995). *A model of human occupation:*

Theory and application (2nd edition). Baltimore: Williams & Wilkins.

COST: $

SAMPLE: PERSONAL CAUSATION

Shows Initiative
Tries New Things
Indicates Pride (verbally or nonverbally)

Social Skills

and

Role Performance

Assessments

☐ Adolescent Role Assessment

AUTHOR: Maureen M. Black

FORMAT: Rating system based on semi-structured interview.

PURPOSE: The instrument assesses past history and present organization of internalized roles. It provides a profile of the adolescent's role development within family, peer, and school situations for clinical use.

POPULATION: Adolescents; developed for use in psychosocial dysfunction. (Sample consisted of 12 in-patients of Neuropsychiatric Institute, UCLA, ages 13 to 17 years, and 28 normal adolescents, ages 13 to 16 years).

SETTING OR POSITION: Not prescribed.

MATERIALS OR TOOLS: Written interview guide for examiner (contains guided questions and scoring).

METHOD: The interview covers 21 topics in 6 areas: childhood play, adolescent socialization in the family, school performance, peer interactions, occupational choice, and work. The interviewer uses the interview guide to direct the conversation, probing in the rating areas until the score (+, 0, -) can be assigned according to written criteria for each topic.

INTERPRETATION: The questions yield both narrative content for treatment planning and an objective rating. The ratings provide a profile of functioning in the six areas.

RELIABILITY: Test–retest reliability based on a small subset of the sample is .91. Item definitions and rating criteria should raise the stability of the tool.

VALIDITY: Content validity is based on literature review.

SOURCES: Black, M.M. Adolescent Role Assessment. *American Journal of Occupational Therapy, 30,* 73–79. (1976)

Black, M.M. (1982). Adolescent Role Assessment. In B. Hemphill (Ed.), *The evaluative process in psychiatric occupational therapy,* Thorofare, NJ: Slack.

COST: ¢

SAMPLE: What games and physical sports did you do as a child?

What kinds of responsibilities did you have at home?

❑ Assessment of Communication & Interaction Skills (ACIS)

AUTHORS: Marcelle Salamy, MS, OTR/L, Sandy Simon, MS, OTR/L, and Gary Kielhofner, DrPH, OTR, FAOTA

FORMAT: Observation-based rating scale.

PURPOSE: ACIS is designed to measure the individual's personal communication and group interaction skills in the course of daily activity. By identifying competencies and deficiencies in this area, it can help in planning intervention. Kielhofner (1995) suggests using the instrument as an aid to clinical judgment due to its early stage of development.

POPULATION: Individuals with psychiatric illness, although appears relevant to a broader population.

SETTING OR POSITION: Designed for use in group settings.

MATERIALS OR TOOLS: Manual, score sheet, and a pencil.

METHOD: ACIS comprises 18 behaviors or action verbs that represent communication and interaction skills in 6 domains: Affective Connectedness, Physicality, Language, Dynamics, Relations, and Information Exchange. One or more subjects are observed in group activity for periods of approximately 30–60 minutes, and then rated on a 4-point scale (4 = competent, 3 = questionable, 2 = ineffective, 1 = deficit). Domain descriptions, definitions of action verbs, and scoring criteria are provided for each item. Descriptive comments may supplement ratings.

INTERPRETATION: At this stage of development, the authors recommend using ACIS informally as a guideline for observation to offer a profile of strengths and weaknesses in communication/interaction. Data may be combined with observations from other settings for a more complete picture.

RELIABILITY: The first version demonstrated low to moderate interrater reliability, resulting in refinement and clarification of the instrument. Research on scoring criteria is ongoing.

VALIDITY: Content validity was established by extensive literature review. Rasch analysis supported a single unidimensional construct of communication and interaction and a hierarchy of the 18 verbs.

SOURCES: Distributed by: Model of Human Occupation Clearinghouse, University of Illinois at Chicago, Department of Occupational Therapy (M/C 811), College of Associated Health Professions, 1919 West Taylor Street, Chicago, IL 60612-7250. Tel: 312-996-6901; Fax: 312-413-0256. (**1989, revised 1993**)

Kielhofner, G. (1995). *A model of human occupation: Theory and application (2nd edition)*. Baltimore: Williams & Wilkins.

COST: $

SAMPLE: *AFFECTIVE/CONNECTEDNESS*

Expresses	1	2	3	4
Gestures	1	2	3	4
Gazes	1	2	3	4

❑ Occupational Role History

AUTHORS: Linda Florey, MA, OTR, and Shirley M. Michelman, MA, OTR

FORMAT: Historical, semistructured interview.

PURPOSE: The Occupational Role History is an abbreviated interview for screening in acute care settings. By collecting data on developmental and recent work–play experiences, it is designed to unfold the development of the individual's occupational roles.

POPULATION: Adults. (Sample consisted of adult psychiatric in- and outpatients at UCLA Neuropsychiatric Institute.)

SETTING OR POSITION: Not prescribed.

MATERIALS OR TOOLS: Interview guidelines.

METHOD: The history is a semistructured interview on occupational choice processes, work experience, sources of work and leisure satisfaction and dissatisfaction, work goals and successes, and characteristics of current work and leisure. Occupational roles are addressed in general, with emphasis on occupational performance. There are 23 questions in the worker/homemaker section, and 11 questions in the school section. The interview requires 1/2 hour.

INTERPRETATION: The data are interpreted according to: role status (rated functional, temporarily impaired, or dysfunctional) and balance (between leisure and occupational roles). Areas for intervention can be identified.

RELIABILITY: No reliability data.

VALIDITY: Face and content validity are apparent, based on theories of occupational development.

SOURCE: Florey, L., & Michelman, S.M. The Occupational Role History: A screening tool for psychiatric occupational therapy. *American Journal of Occupational Therapy, 36*(5), 301–308. (**1982**)

COST: ¢

SAMPLE: "How/why did you choose this occupation?"

"How did you learn the daily routine?"

❒ Role Checklist

AUTHOR: Frances Maag Oakley, MS, OTR/L

FORMAT: Written inventory.

PURPOSE: The checklist assesses productive roles in adult life by indicating the individual's perceptions of his or her past, present, and future roles.

POPULATION: Developed for adult psychiatric patients, but appears appropriate for other adults as well as adolescent and geriatric populations. (Sample administration was completed on undergraduate students.)

SETTING OR POSITION: Not prescribed, although examiner is instructed to remain with subject during test for questions.

MATERIALS OR TOOLS: Questionnaire and pencil (could adapt to oral administration).

METHOD: Ten roles are defined, and the respondent indicates whether he or she has, is, or anticipates being in each role (Part I) and the degree to which the role is valued (Part II). Additional roles can be added by the subject. Points are totaled for each of the following categories: continuous roles, disrupted roles, role changes, past roles, present roles, future roles, not valuable, somewhat valuable, and very valuable. Administration requires approximately 15 minutes.

INTERPRETATION: The checklist helps identify the roles significant to the subject, the motivation to engage in tasks necessary to those roles, and perceptions of role shifting.

RELIABILITY: Test–retest reliability is a median of .82 with a 2-week interval. External confirmation of subject's report of roles is suggested to validate findings.

VALIDITY: Content validity of the taxonomy of roles is based on literature review and consultation with experts.

SOURCES: Obtain from: Frances Oakley, MS, OTR/L, FAOTA, Occupational Therapy Service, National Institutes of Health, Building 10, Room 6S-235, 10 Center Drive MSC 1604, Bethesda, Maryland 20892-1604. (**1984, revised 1988**)

Oakley, F., Kielhofner, G., Barris, R., & Reichler, R.K. (1986). The Role Checklist: Development and empirical assessment of reliability. *Occupational Therapy Journal of Research, 6*(3), 157–169.

SAMPLE: Volunteer: Donating services, <u>at least once a week</u>, to a hospital, school, community, political campaign, and so forth.

COST: ¢

Self-Management

and

Coping Skills

Assessments

❏ AAMR Adaptive Behavior Scale—Residential and Community, Second Edition (ABS-RC:2) and AAMR Adaptive Behavior Scale—School, Second Edition (ABS-S:2)

AUTHORS: Kazuo Nihira, Henry Leland, and Nadine Lambert (School edition: Nadine Lambert, Kazuo Nihira, and Henry Leland)

FORMAT: Standardized behavior rating scales.

PURPOSE: The scales are designed to provide information on the individual's adaptive behavior, that is effectiveness in coping with natural and social demands of the environment. By providing a picture of daily functioning, the test is meant to identify individuals with impairments in adaptive behavior, determine strengths and weaknesses, aid in diagnosis, treatment planning or training, and mark progress. It can be used for clinical or research purposes.

POPULATION: Mentally retarded, emotionally maladjusted, and developmentally disabled children and adults, as well as other handicapped persons, ages 3 years to adult. ABS-S:2 is suitable through age 21, and ABS-RC:2 through age 79. (RC:2 sample consisted of 4,103 individuals with developmental disabilities residing at home or in community facilities in 46 states; S:2 sample consisted of 2,074 mentally retarded persons from 40 states and over 1,000 nonretarded persons in 44 states.)

SETTING OR POSITION: Not prescribed; examiner is advised to observe the subject performing tasks or behaving in as many settings as possible.

MATERIALS OR TOOLS: Manual and scoring booklet, pencil; software scoring and report system is available.

METHOD: The 2-part scale is completed by a caregiver or individuals familiar with the daily behaviors of the subject. Part One consists of 10 domains of personal independence (9 in S:2 edition) organized in developmentally sequenced skills, such as independent func-

tioning, physical development, economic activity, responsibility, and prevocational/vocational activity. Part Two consists of 8 domains of social behavior or maladaptive behavior (7 in the S:2 edition) related to personality and behavior disorders, such as conformity or self-abusive behavior. The rater selects statements most accurately reflecting level of performance or behavior, using item-by-item ratings or interview with a caregiver. Each response has a numerical value (ranging 0–1, 0–2, or 0–3); these are totaled for subdomain and domain scores. Administration requires 15–30 minutes.

INTERPRETATION: Raw scores are recorded and graphed on the Profile/Summary Form, then converted to standard scores, percentiles, and age equivalents using the normative tables. Results are interpreted in terms of Domain Scores, which reflect performance on each adaptive behavior, and Factor Scores for the 5 identified factors (see Validity). Low domain and item scores indicate areas for remediation. Factor scores reflect on the subject's ability to live independently in society. Used with other measures, ABS can assist in diagnosis of mental retardation and other developmental disabilities.

RELIABILITY: Internal consistency of most or all factor scores exceeded .90 (median RC:2=.97), and most or all other scores exceeded .80. Test–retest reliability over a 2-week interval exceeded .80 in all RC:2 scores (most exceeded .90) and nearly all S:2 scores. Interrater reliability for all domain and factor scores ranged from .96–.99 in all but Prevocational/Vocational Activity (RC:2=.83, S:2=.95).

VALIDITY: Factor analysis on the domains identifies 5 factors: personal self-sufficiency, community self-sufficiency, personal-social responsibility, social adjustment, and personal adjustment. Content validity is based on critical review of existing tests and on item analysis. Criterion-related validity is supported by correlation of Part one scores with Vineland Adaptive Behavior Scales and Adaptive Behavior Inventory. Construct validity is evident from the degree of age differentiation in scores, intercorrelations of scores within Parts one and two, correlation of Part one scores with intelligence tests, score differentiation between normal groups and those with developmental disabilities, and correlations of items to domains and factors.

SOURCE: Published by: Pro-Ed, 8700 Shoal Creek Boulevard, Austin, TX 78757-6897. Tel: 512-451-3246; Fax: 800-FXPROED. (**1969, revised 1975, 1993**)

COST: $$

SAMPLE: **Eating in public**
(Circle highest level)

Orders complete meals in restaurants	3
Orders simple meals, like hamburgers and hot dogs	2
Orders single items, e.g., soft drinks, ice cream, donuts, etc. at soda fountain or canteen	1
Does not order at public eating places	0

❒ Coping Inventory

AUTHOR: Shirley Zeitlin, EdD

FORMAT: Rating scale based on observation of behavior.

PURPOSE: This inventory is designed to assess adaptive and maladaptive coping habits, skills, and behaviors that a child uses to manage the world. It can help in classifying handicapped children and in developing intervention plans to improve coping skills in school, daily activities, and the community.

POPULATION: Children ages 3–16; it is contraindicated for children who are too handicapped to learn the behaviors described in the items. (Sample consisted of 1,119 racially diverse children representing typical, handicapped, and environmentally disadvantaged populations, from 16 U.S. locations.) A self-rating format is available for adolescents and adults, ages 15 years and older.

SETTING OR POSITION: Not prescribed, although suggestions for observing the child (e.g., environment, activities) are offered.

MATERIALS OR TOOLS: Manual and Observation form, and a pencil.

METHOD: This 48-item questionnaire is divided into two categories: Coping with Self and Coping with Environment. These are each subdivided into three dimensions to reflect the child's coping style: Productive (using personal resources to achieve results), Active (initiating activity), and Flexible (using a variety and range of strategies). The Inventory observation form is completed by someone familiar with the child or observing the child during three or more 30-minute periods in different situations. The self-rated form is self-administered by the older subject. Each statement is rated from 1–5 reflecting effectiveness of the child's

behavior. Raw scores are totalled for each dimension, and converted to a Self Score and an Environment Score.

INTERPRETATION: The test yields an Adaptive Behavior Index, which indicates how adaptive the child's behavior is and whether intervention is needed. Scores are graphed to illustrate a Coping Profile for each dimension, illustrating the child's specific pattern of behavior. A list of most and least adaptive behaviors is pulled from the high- and low-score items for use in planning intervention. Although a criterion-referenced instrument, results are reported for different sample populations for comparison with the subject's score.

RELIABILITY: Internal consistency among the 6 dimensions ranged from .84–.98, and .97 for the Adaptive Behavior Index. Interrater reliability among 4 trained raters was .92 for the Adaptive Behavior Index of handicapped subjects (ranging .78–.94 for dimension scores) and .895 for nonhandicapped subjects (ranging .78–.89 for dimensions). Factor analysis indicated that the Coping Inventory is a single-factor instrument. Scores of different ethnic groups indicate lack of bias in the test results.

VALIDITY: Content validity is based on extensive literature review and feedback from experts and field test examiners to develop and refine the items and categories. Coping Inventory scores were compared with numerous instruments that assess adaptive behavior, cognitive ability, and life outcomes; the various correlations and noncorrelations are described by the author, including significant correlations between coping and achievement.

SOURCE: Published by: Scholastic Testing Service, Inc. , 480 Meyer Road, Bensenville, IL 60106-1617. Tel: 800-642-6787; Fax: 708-766-8054. (1985)

COST: $

SAMPLE: Coping with Environment: *Productive*

Child is curious (eager to find out about people, objects, situations).

Child is liked and accepted by other children.

❑ Early Coping Inventory

AUTHORS: Shirley Zeitlin, EdD, and G. Gordon Williamson, PhD, OTR, with Margery Szczepanski, MA, OTR

FORMAT: Rating scale based on observation of behavior.

PURPOSE: This instrument was designed to assess the coping-related behaviors used by infants and toddlers in everyday living, specifically the effectiveness, style, and strengths and vulnerabilities in coping skills. It can assist in developing educational and therapeutic intervention to enhance adaptive functioning.

POPULATION: Children ages 4–36 months chronologically, or older children with disabilities who function in that developmental age range. (Sample consisted of 1,035 disabled and 405 nondisabled children from 73 early childhood program sites in the U.S. and Canada.)

SETTING OR POSITION: Not prescribed, although suggestions for observing the child are offered.

MATERIALS OR TOOLS: Manual and Observation form, and a pencil.

METHOD: The Inventory consists of 48 items divided into three categories: Sensorimotor Organization, Reactive Behavior, and Self-Initiated Behavior. It may be administered by professionals or by laypersons under the guidance of a professional, based on prior knowledge and experience or systematic observation (on at least 3 different days) of the child. Each statement of behavior is rated on a 5-point scale ranging from 1 (ineffective coping) to 5 (consistently effective coping), and according to the expectations of the child's developmental age. Raw scores are totalled for each category and converted to an Effectiveness Score on the 1–5 rating scale.

INTERPRETATION: The raw scores and effectiveness scores for each category are combined to yield an Adaptive Behavior Index, which indicates how adaptive the child's behavior is and whether intervention is needed. The categories are graphically illustrated for comparison on a Coping Profile, which depicts the child's specific pattern of behavior. A list of most and least adaptive behaviors is pulled from the high- and low-score items for use in planning intervention.

RELIABILITY: Interrater reliability among 24 trained raters who scored two videotaped subjects twice in a 6-week period, ranged from .80–.94 for the category and Index scores; test–retest reliability was more variable, but with 11 of 16 values showing no significant shift in scoring. Item reliability data is reported in the manual.

VALIDITY: Validity of item content and definitions of coping constructs is demonstrated by literature review and refinement by professionals in educational, psychosocial, and rehabilitative fields as well as by child development experts. The organization and scoring are based on earlier work on the Coping Inventory. Factor analysis lead to the three primary test categories, with four secondary complementary factors.

SOURCE: Published by: Scholastic Testing Service, Inc. , 480 Meyer Road, Bensenville, IL 606106-1617. Tel: 800-642-6787; Fax: 708-766-8054. (**1988**)

COST: $

SAMPLE: <u>Reactive Behavior</u>

Child accepts warmth and support from familiar persons.   1 2 3 4 5

Child reacts to feelings and moods of other people.   1 2 3 4 5

❑ Katz Adjustment Scale

AUTHOR: Martin M. Katz

FORMAT: Paired rating scales.

PURPOSE: These scales attempt to sample areas of behavior considered by clinicians to be indicators of adjustment, using simple perspectives from the subject and an additional social reference. Thus, the language is in simple lay terminology. It provides a picture of social behavior in the community.

POPULATION: Adult prepsychotic (prior to hospitalization) and formerly hospitalized patients. It was designed as a research tool to assess change in patients following intervention and return to the community. (Several studies utilized up to 30 hospitalized psychotic patients, and 404 relatives of institutionalized schizophrenic patients.)

SETTING OR POSITION: Not prescribed.

MATERIALS OR TOOLS: Two test booklets and scoring system.

METHOD: The instrument consists of two sets of five subscales, one set rated by the subject as a self-report and the other rated by a close relative. The five subscales cover: recent symptoms and social behavior (127 items; 55 on self-report), perceptions of level of performance and expectations of performance on socially expected acts (16 items each), level of and satisfaction with free-time activities (23 items each). Approximately 25–45 minutes are needed to rate the items on a 3- or 4-point scale; each item is then scored separately.

INTERPRETATION: The tool yields a profile of adjustment, with two points of view available for comparison.

RELIABILITY: Internal consistency ranges from .61 to .87 among item clusters.

VALIDITY: Preliminary studies indicate scores discriminate between well-adjusted and poorly adjusted groups; concurrent validity is evident in levels of agreement with the ratings of relatives.

SOURCE: Katz, M.M., & Lyerly, S.B. Methods for measuring adjustment and social behavior in the community: I. Rationale, description, discriminative validity and scale development. *Psychological Reports, 13,* 503–535. **(1963)**

COST: ¢

SAMPLE: Scale: Rate from 1 (almost never) to 4 (almost always)

Looks worn out.

Feelings get hurt easily.

❑ Scales of Independent Behavior (SIB)

AUTHORS: Robert H. Bruininks, PhD, Richard W. Woodcock, EdD, Richard F. Weatherman, EdD, and Bradley K. Hill, MA

FORMAT: Structured interview and rating scales.

PURPOSE: This set of tests is a simple yet comprehensive measure of adaptive and problem behaviors. It is designed to provide measurement and program planning information, determine eligibility for services, set goals for Individualized Education or Program Plans, and assist with program evaluation.

POPULATION: Profoundly to mildly handicapped to nonhandicapped children and adults from infancy to maturity. (Normative data are based on a stratified random sample of 1,764 subjects from 3 months to 44 years and from communities throughout the U.S. Special norms are provided for a wide range of intelligence, from severely retarded to gifted, as well as for handicapped and disabled subjects in various educational and residential environments.)

SETTING OR POSITION: Comfortable private interview room with adequate ventilation and lighting, free of distractions and interruptions. Interviewer and respondent are seated at right angles to each other at a table to permit viewing of free-standing test book by both.

MATERIALS OR TOOLS: The interviewer's manual, free-standing flip-page test book, response booklet, and a pencil.

METHOD: SIB consists of 226 items in 14 subscales, organized into four clusters of related subscales: Motor Skills, Social Interaction and Communication Skills, Personal Independence Skills, and Community Independence Skills. Each item consists of a statement of a task necessary for independent function, which is performed without help or supervision. Tasks are arranged in order of development and complexity. The interviewer completes the SIB based on knowledge of the subject's performance or by questioning the subject or a familiar respondent. Items are rated on a 4-point scale, ranging from 0 (NEVER OR RARELY—Even if asked) to 3 (DOES VERY WELL—ALWAYS OR ALMOST ALWAYS—Without being asked). Each subscale requires about 4 minutes, totalling about 1 hour for the complete scale (administration of all subscales is not required). The ratings are totalled for each scale or subscale.

Two 32-item screening versions are also available: the Short Form Scale consists of discriminating items from all 14 subscales, and the Early Development Scale assesses very young (birth–2 1/2 years) or severely handicapped children. They require 10–15 minutes each.

In addition, a Problem Behaviors Scale consists of examples of problem behaviors in 8 categories (e.g., Hurtful to Self, Destructive to Property) and requires about 5–10 minutes to administer. The respondent indicates the presence of the behavior, frequency (from 1—less than once a month, to 5—1 or more times an hour), severity, and how it is usually managed.

INTERPRETATION: Several types of scores are available to facilitate interpretation. Normative scores include age scores, percentile ranks, and standard scores. Instructional Functioning scores describe the level of performance by the subject, for planning instruction or training activities. Adjusted adaptive behavior functioning scores are compared statistically to the Woodcock-Johnson Psycho-Educational Battery norms in order to compare with others of same age and intelligence. Scores from the Problem Behaviors Scale can be combined into four broader maladaptive behavior indices to summarize the subject's problem behavior. All scores can be graphed on Percentile Rank Profiles, a Subscale Profile, a

Training Implications Profile, and a Problem Behaviors Profile.

RELIABILITY: Items and subscales were developed through Rasch Analysis. Split-half reliability coefficients were mostly in the high .70–.80's for subtests and high .80–.90's for clusters; low coefficients resulting from items that had not been learned by the younger subjects or had been mastered by the older do not reflect on internal consistency, the authors state. Test–retest reliability within a 4-week interval ranged from .87–.96 for Full Scale and Short Form and .75–.86 for combined ages in Problem Behaviors. Interrater reliability was .99–1.0 for all Full Scale and most Problem Behavior scores, with remaining correlations in the .90s.

VALIDITY: Construct validity studies confirm adaptive behavior to be developmental in nature. They discriminate among more severely handicapped and non-handicapped people, with fewer differences among mildly handicapped and nonhandicapped; this finding was duplicated with the Maladaptive Behavior Indexes. There was strong agreement between the short scales and Full Scale scores (.80s). Criterion-related studies demonstrated correlations between scores on SIB and Adaptive Behavior Scale (School Edition), Woodcock-Johnson Broad Cognitive Ability, Quay Problem Behavior Checklist, and parent/teacher evaluations. SIB scores correctly classified subjects for employment training and school placement. Content validity is based on surveys of existing theories, taxonomies, and tests of adaptive and problem behaviors.

SOURCES: Published by: The Riverside Publishing Company, 8420 Bryn Mawr Avenue, Chicago, IL 60603. Tel: 800-767-8378. (**1984 by DLM**)

Bruininks, R.H., Woodcock, R.W., Weatherman, R.F., & Hill, B.K. (1985). *Development and standardization of the scales of independent behavior.* Chicago: Riverside Publishing Co.

COST: $$$; computer scoring program $$$. $—*Development and Standardization of the Scales of Independent Behavior*

SAMPLE: Home/Community Orientation

Crosses nearby residential streets, roads, and unmarked intersections alone.

Finds planned destination, when confused, by asking directions, telephoning for help, or otherwise regaining direction.

❑ Street Survival Skills Questionnaire (SSSQ)

AUTHORS: Lawrence McCarron, PhD and Dan Linkenhoker, PhD

FORMAT: Norm-based pictorial multiple choice test.

PURPOSE: The SSSQ was designed to assess the level of community-related adaptive skills for prevocational evaluation. It provides an objective measure of specific aspects of adaptive behavior, a baseline to determine the effects of training, and a prediction for community living and vocational placement.

POPULATION: Special education students as well as children, adolescents, and adults with mental retardation or other physical, mental, or developmental disabilities. (Norms are available for neuropsychologically disabled adults ages 15–55, based on a sample of 500; normal adolescents and adults ages 16–40, based on a sample of 200; and normal children ages 9.5–15, based on a sample of 271.)

SETTING OR POSITION: The evaluator sits opposite the subject with the page of plates in front of the subject.

MATERIALS OR TOOLS: Carrying case includes binder containing 9 volumes of picture plates, manual, Curriculum Guides for the SSSQ, scoring forms, and master planning charts. A computer program is available for reporting results.

METHOD: SSSQ consists of 9 sections, each relating to a specific area of adaptive behavior: Basic Concepts, Functional Signs, Tools, Domestic Management, Health and Safety, Public Services, Time, Money, and Measurement. Every section contains 24 pages, each with 4 pictures related to daily living tasks and a relevant question on the facing page. The examiner asks the question and the subject indicates (orally or by pointing) the correct response picture. Raw scores are totalled

for each component; these are converted to scaled scores and may be plotted on the Score Form Profile and Master Planning Chart for an overview of results. The large print and graphics are visible to the visually impaired, and instructions for the hearing impaired (in American Sign Language) are available. Administration requires 30–45 minutes.

INTERPRETATION: SSSQ provides an estimate of community and living skills, as well as an expected level of vocational placement. Scaled scores may be compared to the norms as well as to each other to indicate relative strengths and needs for the Individual Education/ Program Plan. Conversion tables are available to convert raw scores into a Survival Skills Quotient for comparison with IQ and with expected level of vocational programming (for adult subjects). Curriculum Guides are available for intervention purposes, providing teaching strategies, activities, and performance criteria.

RELIABILITY: Internal consistency was demonstrated by a total test reliability coefficient of .97 for the total score, and a range of .68–.96 on the subtests. Test–retest reliability ranged from .81–.95 (subtests) and .99 for the total.

VALIDITY: Content validity is based on item analysis by literature review, interviews with staff, analysis of behaviors, and statistical analysis of items, to develop an adequate sample of the content area. Factor analysis of the 9 subtests indicated one adaptive behavior factor related to communication that was shared among all subtests. SSSQ scores correlated with Peabody Picture Vocabulary Test IQ scores in a diverse developmentally disabled group, and specific SSSQ scores correlated moderately with reading scores, supporting construct validity. SSSQ also correlates with measures of vocational competency and adaptive communications behavior. Finally SSSQ is used as a component of the

McCarron-Dial System to predict work potential and placement for neuropsychologically disabled adults.

SOURCE: Produced by: McCarron-Dial Systems, PO Box 45628, Dallas, TX 75245. Tel: 214-247-5945. **(1979, revised in 1993)**

COST: $$$; $$$ for computer program.

SAMPLE: Functional Signs and Symbols

Which light tells you to go?

Which sign shows a safe place to cross the street?

❏ Vineland Adaptive Behavior Scales, Revised (VABS)

AUTHORS: Sara S. Sparrow, David A. Balla, and Domenic V. Cicchetti

FORMAT: Standardized performance scales, using semi-structured interview (interview editions) or questionnaire (classroom edition).

PURPOSE: A revision of the Vineland Social Maturity Scale (1935, 1965), this instrument is designed to assess an individual's performance of the daily activities necessary for personal and social sufficiency, that is, to take care of oneself and get along with others.

POPULATION: Individuals from birth to adulthood. (The norms for the survey and expanded forms are based on a national sample of 48,000 subjects from birth to 18 years, 11 months. The classroom edition is standardized for ages 3 to 12 years, 11 months.) Supplementary norms for handicapped groups were obtained from samples of mentally retarded, visually impaired, hearing impaired, and emotionally disturbed individuals. It is also recommended for low-functioning adults.

SETTING OR POSITION: Quiet room with comfortable chairs, spacious enough for interviewer, materials, and respondent; subject or other individuals should not be present.

MATERIALS OR TOOLS: Each edition has its own manual and record booklet or, for the expanded form, an item booklet, score summary, and profile booklet, plus program planning report and pencil.

METHOD: This tool measures adaptive behavior in four domains: communication, daily living skills, socialization, and motor skills. In addition, a maladaptive behavior domain may be used to identify undesirable behaviors that interfere with function (for subjects 5 years or older); it consists of two parts, for minor and for serious behaviors. There are three versions. (1) The

interview edition, survey form, contains 297 items and requires 20–60 minutes to administer. (2) The interview edition, expanded form, contains 577 items (including the survey items) and requires 60–90 minutes to administer. It can be used independently or to supplement the assessment of areas found to be weak by the survey form; both are given by a trained interviewer to a parent or primary caregiver. While the survey form offers a general assessment, the expanded form is more comprehensive and offers a systematic basis for treatment planning. (3) The classroom edition consists of 244 items in questionnaire format which can be completed by the classroom teacher in about 20 minutes.

The items are arranged in age order, and items appropriate to the subject's chronological or mental age are administered. The interview consists of general questions designed to elicit specific information on what the subject typically does (rather than *can* do). Each item is scored 2 (indicating satisfactory and habitual performance), 1 (emerging or partial performance), or 0 (cannot or does not perform). Maladaptive behaviors are also scored from 2 (behavior usually present) to 0.

INTERPRETATION: Raw scores are converted to standard scores for each domain, plus an adaptive behavior composite score, with age equivalents, national percentile ranks, and adaptive level interpretations for both. Norms and supplementary norms for 7 handicapping conditions are available for comparison. Results can assist with diagnosis of mental retardation, educational placement, planning intervention, following progress, and comparison of performance among domains. Extensive guidelines for interpretation are offered.

RELIABILITY: Split-half reliability median coefficients were in the .80–.90s for domain and adaptive behavior composite scores and .60–.90s for subdomain scores (higher for supplementary norm groups). Test–retest reliability with a 2- to 4-week interval was very good, with most coefficients in the .80–90s for domain and composite survey socres. Interrater reliability for survey domain and composite scores was in the .70s except for Socialization (.62).

VALIDITY: Content validity is supported by thorough review of literature and other adaptive behavior scales, and by subsequent field testing of items and the national standardization process. Construct validity was demonstrated by the developmental progression of scores (confirming age-related adapative behavior); by factor analysis supporting the organization of domains and subdomains; and by score profiles differentiating among the 7 supplementary norm groups of handicapped individuals and the general norm group. Criterion-

related validity is supported by correlation of .55 between the Vineland composite score with the original Vineland scores and by low correlation between the Vineland and intelligence tests (confirming they are different areas of function).

SOURCE: Published by: American Guidance Service, Inc., Publishers' Building, Circle Pines, MN 55014. Tel: 800-328-2560; Fax: 612-786-9077. (**1984–Survey; 1985–Classroom**)

COST: $

SAMPLE: Communication Domain:
Turns eyes and head toward sound .(Receptive)
Says at least 50 recognizable words. (Expressive)
Addresses envelope completely. (Written)

PERFORMANCE CONTEXTS

Temporal Aspects/Disability Status

Assessments

❑ Disability Questionnaire

AUTHORS: Martin Roland, MA, MRCP, MRCGP and Richard Morris, MSc

FORMAT: Self-rated questionnaire.

PURPOSE: This short and simple questionnaire was developed to measure self-rated disability due to back pain in order to serve as an outcome measure for evaluation of intervention. It is sensitive enough to distinguish between spontaneous improvement and treatment results.

POPULATION: Individuals with low back pain. (Sample consisted of 230 back pain patients, ages 16–64 years, registered with a group practice during 1 calendar year.)

SETTING OR POSITION: Not prescribed.

MATERIALS OR TOOLS: Questionnaire and pencil.

METHOD: The questionnaire consists of 24 descriptive statements covering a range of daily living aspects and derived from the Sickness Impact Profile. The subject checks those statements that pertain to himself or herself "today." It is completed in about 5 minutes and yields a single score by totalling 1 point for each statement checked.

INTERPRETATION: The score ranges from 0 (no disability) to 24 (severe disability). Poor outcome was defined for the study as a score of 14 or more. (The mean score of the sample population presenting to a family practice was 11.4.)

RELIABILITY: Test–retest reliability with same-day retesting yielded a correlation of .91 (.83 agreement per cent coefficient indicated the degree to which same individual items were checked).

VALIDITY: Agreement between the questionnaire and a 6-point pain rating scale was good; questionnaire score was a more discriminating indicator of outcome than the pain rating scale due to its significant relationship to 14 clinical features found by examination of the patients.

SOURCE: Published in: Roland, M., & Morris, R. A study of the natural history of back pain Part I: Development of a reliable and sensitive measure of disability in low-back pain. *Spine, 8,* 141–144. (**1983**)

COST: ¢

SAMPLE: I stay at home most of the time because of my back.

I change position frequently to try and get my back comfortable.

❏ National Institutes of Health Activity Record (ACTRE)

AUTHOR: Gloria Furst, OTR/L, MPH

FORMAT: Questionnaire based on 24-hour log.

PURPOSE: Based on the Model of Human Occupation, ACTRE provides a detailed account of how the subject spends time, as well as the impact of symptoms on daily performance, interests, and habits. It can be used in treatment planning, documenting change, and tracking patients over the course of an illness.

POPULATION: Designed for patients with rheumatoid arthritis, it is applicable to adolescents and adults with a variety of diagnoses, including progressive neuromuscular and neurological conditions. (A sample of 21 subjects with rheumatoid arthritis participated in the validation study.)

SETTING OR POSITION: Not prescribed.

MATERIALS OR TOOLS: Activity Record log, instructions, and a pencil. Use of a computer spreadsheet for scoring is now recommended; this can be obtained by sending a disc to the author (see Source) for a copy of the spreadsheet (Microsoft Excel program for Windows or Mac).

METHOD: The Activity Record consists of a written log broken down into 1/2-hour time slots. For a period of 2 days, subjects write what they were doing during each time slot, the level of energy required (standing, sitting, or lying down activity), and which of nine categories the activity falls into (e.g., rest, self-care, preparation, or planning). Finally, each activity is rated on a 4-point scale according to questions about skill, enjoyment, fatigue, etc. The log should be completed at three points during each recorded day to ensure accuracy. The raw data are converted into frequency and percent of waking hours and recorded on the Summary Form.

INTERPRETATION: The ACTRE summary provides quantifiable information on roles and habits regarding sleep and activity patterns, occurrence of symptoms, and motivation for activities. Results yield information on the appropriateness of time spent in various roles, balance of activity and rest, relationship of symptoms to activity, and the subject's perceptions of performance. These data assist with treatment planning and detects changes resulting from disease or intervention.

RELIABILITY: As activities and the state of the individual are variable, the Record is not expected to be stable on different days.

VALIDITY: ACTRE correlates well with other measures of pain, fatigue, and ADL performance. It is unique in identifying specific daily activities likely to cause symptoms.

SOURCE: Available from the author: Gloria Furst, MPH, OTR, Department of Rehabilitation Medicine, Warren Grant Magnuson Clinical Center, National Institutes of Health, Building 10, Room 6S-235, 10 Center Drive MSC 1604, Bethesda, MD 20892-1604. Tel: 301-402-3017.

Gerber, L., & Furst, G. (1992). Validation of the NIH activity record: A quantitative measure of life activities. *Arthritis Care Research, 5,* 81–86.

COST: ¢

SAMPLE: For Me This Activity is

> 1=Not Meaningful
> 2=Slightly Meaningful
> 3=Meaningful
> 4=Very Meaningful

❏ Oswestry Low Back Pain Disability Questionnaire

AUTHORS: Jeremy C. T. Fairbank, FRCS, Jean B. Davies, MSCP, DipPhysEd, Judith Couper, MBAOT, and John P. O'Brien, PhD, FRCS

FORMAT: Questionnaire.

PURPOSE: This questionnaire is designed to measure level of function as an indication of disability, that is, the limitations of performance when compared to that of a fit person. It provides a subjective assessment of activities of daily living relevant to the low back pain population.

POPULATION: Individuals with low back pain. (Developed at an orthopedic hospital in England, and validated on a group of 25 patients suffering from their first incidence of low back pain.)

SETTING OR POSITION: Not prescribed.

MATERIALS OR TOOLS: Questionnaire printed on colored paper; a pencil.

METHOD: The questionnaire is divided into 10 sections: pain intensity, personal care, lifting, walking, sitting, standing, sleeping, sex life, social life, and travelling. Each section contains 6 graded statements describing degrees of difficulty, as defined by amount of pain experienced. The subject checks the statement in each section that most accurately describes his or her limitations. The statements are scored on a 0–5 scale, 5 representing the greatest disability, and the scores are totalled. It is completed in 3–5 minutes, or more if reading difficulty necessitates assistance.

INTERPRETATION: The score is expressed as a percentage: 0–20% indicates minimal disability, 20–40% moderate disability, 40–60% severe disability, 60–80% crippled, and 80–100% bed-bound or exaggerating the symptoms. Scores are used as a guide to treatment planning.

RELIABILITY: Test–retest reliability of .99 was found upon completion of the questionnaire on 2 consecutive days. Good internal consistency was reported, as mean scores of individual activity sections tended to rise with the mean score of the pain section.

VALIDITY: Concurrent validity is demonstrated in a study of patients with their first incidence of low back pain, in which mean scores improved over a 2- to 3-week period of expected spontaneous recovery.

SOURCE: Published in: Fairbank, J.C.T., Davies, J.B., Couper, J., & O'Brien, J.P. The Oswestry Low Back Pain Disability Questionnaire. *Physiotherapy*, 66, 271–273. (**1980**)

COST: ¢

SAMPLE: Lifting

[_] I can lift heavy weights without extra pain.

[_] I can lift heavy weights but it gives extra pain. ...

[_] I cannot lift or carry anything at all.

❑ Sickness Impact Profile™ (SIP)

AUTHORS: Marilyn Bergner, PhD, Ruth A. Bobbit, PhD, Betty S. Gilson, MD, and others who participated in the development of SIP

FORMAT: Self-rated checklist.

PURPOSE: This behaviorally based measure of perceived health status was developed to detect changes or differences in health status that occur over time or between groups. By determining the impact of illness on everyday activity, it is intended to measure the effects or outcomes of health care for the purpose of evaluation, program planning, and policy formation.

POPULATION: Broadly applicable across types and severities of illness. (Field trials were conducted on a stratified random sample of 696 prepaid group practice enrollees and 199 sick patients of a medical clinic, with additional samples of patients with hyperthyroidism, rheumatoid arthritis, and hip replacements.)

SETTING OR POSITION: Not prescribed.

MATERIALS OR TOOLS: Checklist, *User's Manual and Interpretation Guide* (in press), and a pencil.

METHOD: The SIP contains 136 statements about health-related dysfunction in 12 areas of everyday activity: sleep and rest, eating, work, home management, recreation and pastimes, ambulation, mobility, body care and movement, social interaction, alertness behavior, emotional behavior, and communication. The categories fall into 2 dimensions: physical and psychosocial. The questionnaire is best administered to the subject for self-administration, the subject checking those statements that describe him or her on a given day. Administration requires 20–30 minutes and yields overall, category, and dimension scores. A Spanish translation is available. In addition, a modified version was developed for the low back pain population (Deyo, 1986).

INTERPRETATION: Total score offers an outcome measure for health care planning and evaluation. Category and dimension scores present a profile of self-perception of sickness.

RELIABILITY: Test–retest reliability was .97 for interviewer administration, significantly higher than interviewer-delivered self-administration (.87). Internal consistency was .94.

VALIDITY: Construct and criterion-related validity were supported by correlations of SIP scores with self-assessment of dysfunction (.69), self-assessment of sickness (.63), with National Health Interview Survey index (.55), and with clinician assessment of dysfunction (.50) more than with clinician assessment of sickness (.40). A method of profile and pattern analysis was developed to describe and assess similarities and differences among groups.

SOURCES: Copyrighted by: Johns Hopkins University, all rights reserved, Health Sciences Research and Development Center, 624 N. Broadway, Room 647, Baltimore, MD 21205-1901. **(1977)**

For more information, contact: Sickness Impact Profile, Johns Hopkins University, School of Public Health, Department of Health Policy and Management, 624 N. Broadway, Room 647, Baltimore, MD 21205-1901/

Bergner, M., Bobbitt, R.A., Carter, W.B., & Gilson, B.S. (1981). The Sickness Impact Profile: Development and final revision of a health status measure. *Medical Care*, XIX, 787–805.

Deyo, R.A. (1986). Comparative validity of the Sickness Impact Profile and shorter scales for functional assessment on low-back pain. *Spine*, 11, 951–954.

COST: ¢

SAMPLE: I do not speak clearly when I am under stress

I am not doing any of my usual physical recreation or activities

Environmental

Assessments

❏ Environmental Response Inventory

AUTHOR: George E. McKechnie

FORMAT: True–false checklist.

PURPOSE: This tool is designed to assess the way individuals relate to their environments (regarding attitudes, sentiments, beliefs, and values) and their preferences in choosing environments. It can be used to predict environment-related behavior and is suggested to indicate environmental dispositions correlating with personality patterns. In its current state of validation, the instrument is meant for research use only.

POPULATION: Older adolescents and adults. (Preliminary norms available for adults and college students.)

SETTING OR POSITION: A quiet place to work.

MATERIALS OR TOOLS: Questionnaire, pencil.

METHOD: The inventory addresses 11 dimensions, although the 5 male-linked dimensions are segregated from the 6 female-linked. Some of these dimensions include concerns with conservation, fear of environmental dangers, preferences for urban or pastoral settings, and preferences for stimulation. The scale consists of 218 true–false questions regarding the individual's typical behavior. It is self-administered, individually or in groups, requiring 25–30 minutes.

INTERPRETATION: The inventory yields a profile of preferences for relating to the environment.

RELIABILITY: The mean split-half reliability coefficients are .80 for both samples. Mean test–retest reliability is .86 for all 9 scales. The author cautions that users be well-versed in psychological testing.

VALIDITY: Concurrent validity is suggested by preliminary research comparing the instrument with personal-ity measures, sample behaviors, and demographic variables.

SOURCE: Published by: Consulting Psychologists Press, 3803 E. Bayshore Road, PO Box 10096, Palo Alto, CA 94303. Tel: 800-624-1765; Fax: 415-969-8608. **(1974)**

COST: $

SAMPLE: I occasionally take a walk in the rain just for the experience.

I would enjoy living in a modern, high-rise apartment.

❑ Home Observation for Measurement of the Environment (HOME)

AUTHOR: Dr. Bettye Caldwell

FORMAT: Checklist based on observation and interview.

PURPOSE: The inventory investigates the stimulation potential of the early developmental environment by examining the daily transactions and activities occurring in the homes of young children. By assessing the quality and quantity of social, emotional, and cognitive support available in the environment, assets and liabilities may be identified. It is intended primarily as a screening instrument.

POPULATION: Homes of families with children ranging in age from birth to 6 years; there are two versions of the inventory, one for homes of infants and toddlers (birth to 3 years), and one for homes of preschool children (3 to 6 years). (Samples are based on over 400 families from Little Rock, Arkansas.)

SETTING OR POSITION: Child's home with child awake and present.

MATERIALS OR TOOLS: Observation and interview forms, manual, and a pencil.

METHOD: The two versions of the HOME are similar; Infants and Toddlers Scale consists of 45 items divided into six subscales. The Preschool Scale contains 55 yes-no questions divided into eight subscales of environmental properties (human and nonhuman). Information is gathered during an observation in the child's home followed by an interview with a parent. Administration takes approximately 1 hour.

INTERPRETATION: The instrument yields a total score indicating absence or presence of supports in the home, and eight subscale scores delineating these supports more specifically.

RELIABILITY: Infants and Toddlers: internal consistency (.84 total scale, .39 to .73 for subscales) was judged acceptable for its length; test–retest reliability at 6-month, 12-month, and 24-month age levels were reported good (.24 to .77 for subscales).

Preschool: internal consistency was good (.93 total scale, .53 to .83 range for subscales); test–retest reliability varied widely over an 18-month interval (.05 to .70).

VALIDITY: Extensive validity studies demonstrate correlations between test scores and other measures of early cognitive development and IQ. Infant and Toddler scores are predictive of later IQ levels (retardation versus average/above-average); construct validity is apparent in discriminating between normal and at-risk homes.

SOURCE: Obtain from: Lorraine Coulson, CRTL Room 205, University of Arkansas at Little Rock, 2801 S. University, Little Rock, AR 72204. Tel: 501-569-3423; Fax: 501-569-8694. (**revised 1984**)

COST: $

SAMPLE: Language stimulation:

Parent teaches child some simple manners. (yes/no)

Child is permitted some choice in mealtime menus. (yes/no)

❏ Social Climate Scale: Family Environment Scale (Third Edition) (FES)

AUTHORS: Rudolf H. Moos, PhD and Bernice S. Moos

FORMAT: True–false questionnaire.

PURPOSE: One of 10 Social Climate Scales, the FES examines the social-environmental characteristics of families, contrasting parent and child perceptions to formulate clinical case descriptions, assess family strengths and problems, and identify important issues for family treatment. It can also be used to train therapists in family interactions and influences.

POPULATION: Adolescents and adults, ages 11 years and over; children's version is used for children ages 5–11. (Sample consisted of over 1,000 people in 285 diverse families, with additional respondents contributing to the alternate forms.)

SETTING OR POSITION: Quiet, comfortable, well-lit room with space for each respondent to work.

MATERIALS OR TOOLS: Test manual, test booklet, answer sheets, profile forms, scoring key, and pencils.

METHOD: The FES consists of 90 items in 10 subscales, which are organized according to three basic dimensions: Relationship (Cohesion, Expressiveness, and Conflict), Personal Growth (Independence, Achievement Orientation, Intellectual-Cultural Orientation, Active-Recreational Orientation, and Moral-Religious Emphasis), and System Maintenance (Organization and Control). There are three alternate forms of the test available: The Real Form that measures people's perceptions of their nuclear family, the Ideal Form that allows respondents to describe the kind of family they prefer, and the Expectations Form which is useful for new family situations or changes in circumstances such as a major illness. Items consist of true–false statements that are then scored by a scoring template. For each subscale, raw scores are added up and converted to standard

scores. The Children's Version is a 30-item pictorial adaptation that uses cartoon figures to represent the relevant characteristics. Administration requires 15–20 minutes; all members of a family may be tested simultaneously.

INTERPRETATION: The FES yields standard scores that may be displayed as individual and family profiles. These profiles are compared with the normative group, as well as comparing family members' perceptions and interactions with each other. A typology of family environments is offered, identifying seven family types for use in formulating prognoses and interventions. The publisher will provide a narrative report interpreting the results upon request.

RELIABILITY: Internal consistency ranged from .61–.78 for the 10 subscales. Test–retest reliability of the 10 subscale scores over an 8-week interval ranged from .68–.86, .54–.91 over a 4-month interval, and .52–.89 over 12 months. Mean profile stability correlations were .78 (4-month) and .71 (12-month).

VALIDITY: Content and face validity are based on examination by independent raters and by item-to-item and item-to-scale correlations to define the constructs and select items to fit them. Construct validity studies are described that examine the relationships between family characteristics and perceptions, family roles and social functioning, and between reports by family members and independent raters. Factor analytic studies yielded little agreement on the factor structure. Additional research demonstrates discrimination by FES among families, associations between family climate and life transitions and crises, impact of family environment on members, and relationship of family characteristics to treatment processes and outcome. Many other research applications are described in the manual.

SOURCE: Published by: Consulting Psychologists Press, 577 College Avenue, Palo Alto, CA 94306. Tel: 800-624-1765; Fax: 415-969-8608. (**1981, revised 1986, 1994**)

COST: $

SAMPLE: Getting ahead in life is very important in our family.

We rarely go to lectures, plays or concerts.

Friends often come over for dinner or to visit.

Social Climate Scales: Ward Atmosphere Scale (WAS) and Community-Oriented Programs Environment Scale (COPES)

AUTHOR: Rudolf Moos

FORMAT: True–false test.

PURPOSE: These scales assess the psychosocial atmosphere of various environments as they are perceived by its inhabitants: staff and clients. Comparisons can be made between the inhabitants' ideal preferences and actual perceptions, identifying areas for change.

POPULATION: Clients and/or staff of the setting to be assessed. WAS: psychiatric hospital ward. (Norms are based on a sample of 160 wards selected in U.S.) COPES: community psychiatric programs. (Norms are based on a sample consisting of 54 programs in the U.S. and 20 in the U.K., such as day care and halfway houses).

SETTING OR POSITION: Quiet, comfortable, well-lighted room with ample space to work.

MATERIALS OR TOOLS: Manual, test booklet, scoring key, and pencil with eraser.

METHOD: The WAS and COPES scales consist of 10 subscales representing dimensions of relationships, programming, and administration (e.g., involvement, autonomy, practical orientation). They each consist of 100 items but have 40-item short-form alternates. The items are descriptive statements about the environment. The respondent answers true or false: whether it is characteristic of the actual and/or ideal program (Real Form and Ideal Form) or the expectations of a program not yet begun (Expectations Form). The scales yield raw and standard scores for the 10 dimensions. They are generally administered to groups.

INTERPRETATION: A profile of scores for the 10 dimensions can be compared to norms. Client perceptions can be compared to staff perceptions in evaluating the environment, determining the inhabitants' values, monitoring program changes, and improving the program.

RELIABILITY: WAS internal consistency is acceptable (mean .66 for patients and .71 for staff). Test–retest reliability with 1-week intervals is reported adequate (.68 to .83 range for the subscales). COPES internal consistency is good (mean .79 for members and .78 for staff) and supports 10 distinct but related dimensions. Test–retest reliability averaged .81–.98 for members and .81–.60 for staff over intervals ranging from 4–6 months to 24 months.

VALIDITY: Numerous studies are described that compare treatment milieus and their impact on client behavior, the effects of client perceptions of the environment, and the connections between treatment environments and outcomes. These studies support construct, concurrent, and predictive validity.

SOURCE: Published by: Mind Garden, Inc., PO Box 60669, Palo Alto, CA 94306. Tel: 415-424-8493; Fax: 415-424-0475. **(1974, second editions 1988)**

COST: $ for each.

SAMPLE: 1. New treatment approaches are often tried on this ward.

2. This place usually looks a little messy.

Additional Resources

❐ Additional Resources

Other sources of instrument titles with varying descriptive and critical information include the following (see also Notes section):

- AOTA Special Interest Groups each publish a list of evaluation tools; contact the Practice Division of the AOTA.
- Publishers known to publish tests relevant to occupational therapy; write to them for catalogs (see selected list in Index of Publishers).
- Most general textbooks in occupational therapy contain chapters on assessment and assessment tools applicable to different specialties.
- Most graduate schools in occupational therapy keep copies of theses and dissertations in their library collections; access to unpublished manuscripts and availability for purchase vary with the institution.
- AOTA has produced a 49-minute videotape entitled Principles of Measurement (1988) in which Bette Bonder lectures on standardized test and measurement terminology.
- Journal searches reveal newly developed short tests and new research on existing tests.
- Kielhofner (1995) provides an appendix of 12 instruments developed for the Model of Human Occupation.
- Hemphill's texts (1982, 1988, and pending in 1996) offer expanded, in-depth descriptions of evaluations for use in psychiatry, including discussion of the evaluative process and research analysis.
- Cole et al. (1994) offer a rationale and description of outcome measures using the International Classification for Impairment, Disability and Handicap, and include summaries of 60 rehabilitation measures.
- Denton's workbook (1987) offers practical exercises for the student of psychiatric assessment.
- Clark and Allen (1985) contains three chapters describing basic methods of pediatric assessment and screening and reviewing specific evaluation instruments.
- King-Thomas and Hacker (1987) describe and compare over sixty pediatric tests with additional chapters on examiner responsibilities, instrument selection, and the use of standardized tests for the physically handicapped child.
- Reilly (1974) contains methodologies for evaluating and studying play behavior.
- Parham and Fazio (in press) contains updated information on play.
- Robinson and Shaver' product (1973) contains several-page descriptions of over 120 tests on different aspects of social and personality traits (e.g., values, self-esteem).
- The Mental Measurements Yearbooks contain test information, critical reviews and comprehensive bibliographies on thousands of tests published in any English-speaking country.
- Tests in Print contains a comprehensive index of all tests published in English in the fields of education, psychology and industry.

(Note: the latter two sources were formerly known by the Buros Institute that published all early editions up to the 1980s.)

References

❒ References

Allen, C.K. (1985). *Occupational therapy for psychiatric diseases: Measurement and management of cognitive disabilities*. Boston: Little, Brown.

American Educational Research Association, American Psychological Association, National Council on Measurement in Education. (1985). *Standards for educational and psychological testing*. Washington, DC: Author.

American Occupational Therapy Association. (1994). Uniform terminology for occupational therapy—Third edition. *American Journal of Occupational Therapy, 48,* 1047–1054.

Anastasi, A. (1988). *Psychological testing* (6th ed.). New York: MacMillan.

Benson, J., & Clark, F. (1982). A guide for instrument development and validation. *American Journal of Occupational Therapy, 32,* 789–800.

Bonder, B. (1993). Issues in assessment of psychosocial components of function. *American Journal of Occupational Therapy, 47,* 211–216.

Bonder, B. (1985). Standardized assessments: Ethical principles for use. *American Journal of Occupational Therapy, 39,* 473–474.

Bruininks, R.H., Woodcock, R.W., Hill, B.K., & Weatherman, R.F. (1985). *Development and standardization of the Scales of Independent Behavior*. Chicago: Riverside Publishing.

Clark, P.N., & Allen, A.S. (1985). *Occupational therapy for children*. Princeton, NJ: Mosby.

Cole, B., Finch, E., Gowland, C., & Mayo, N. (1994). In J. Basmajian (Ed.), *Physical rehabilitation outcome measures*. Toronto, Ontario: Canadian Physiotherapy Association.

Conoley, J.C., & Kramer, J.J. (Eds.). (1989). *The tenth mental measurements yearbook*. Lincoln, NE: University of Nebraska Press.

Cronbach, L.J. (1970). *Essentials of psychological testing* (3rd ed.). New York: Harper & Row.

Denton, P.L. (1987) *Psychiatric occupational therapy: A workbook of practical skills*. Boston: Little, Brown.

Dunn, W. (Ed.). (1991). *Pediatric occupational therapy*. Thorofare, NJ: Slack.

Fox, D.J. (1969). *The research process in education*. New York: Holt, Rinehart, and Winston.

Freeman, F.S. (1962). *Theory and practice of psychological testing* (3rd ed.). New York: Holt, Rinehart & Winston.

Hasselkus, B.R., & Safrit, M.J. (1976). Measurement in occupational therapy. *American Journal of Occupational Therapy, 30,* 429–436.

Hemphill, B. (Ed.). (1982). *The evaluative process in psychiatric occupational therapy*. Thorofare, NJ: Slack.

Hemphill, B. (Ed.). (1988). *Mental health assessment in occupational therapy*. Thorofare, NJ: Slack.

Hopkins, H.L., & Smith, H.D. (1993). *Willard and Spackman's occupational therapy* (8th ed.). Philadelphia: Lippincott.

Kielhofner, G. (1995). *A model of human occupation: Theory and application (2nd ed.)*. Baltimore: Williams & Wilkins.

King-Thomas, L., & Hacker, B.J. (Eds.). (1987). *A therapist's guide to pediatric assessment*. Boston: Little, Brown.

Maurer, P., Barris, R., Bonder, B., & Gillette, N. (1984). Hierarchy of competencies relating to the use of standardized instruments and evaluation techniques by occupational therapists. *American Journal of Occupational Therapy, 38,* 803–804.

Miller, L.J. (Ed.). (1989). *Developing norm-referenced standardized tests*. Binghamton, NY: Haworth.

Murphy, L. (Ed.). (1994). *Tests in print IV*. Lincoln, NE: University of Nebraska Press.

Ottenbacher, K.J., & Tomchek, S.D. (1993). Reliability analysis in therapeutic research: Practice and procedures. *American Journal of Occupational Therapy, 47,* 10–16.

Parham, D., & Fazio, L. (Eds.). (in press). *Play: A clinical focus in occupational therapy for children*. St. Louis, MO: Mosby Yearbooks.

Reilly, M. (Ed.). (1974). *Play as exploratory learning: Studies of curiosity behavior*. Beverly Hills, CA: Sage.

Robinson, J.P., & Shaver, P.R. (1973). *Measures of social psychological attitudes*. Ann Arbor, MI: Institute of Social Research.

Synder, S., & Sheehan, R. (1992). Research methods: The Rasch measurement model: An introduction. *Journal of Early Intervention, 16*(1), 87–95.

Tarczan, C. (1962). *An educator's guide to psychological tests*. Springfield, IL: Charles C. Thomas.

Index of Publishers

❑ Index of Publishers

Academic Therapy Publications (**pp. 102, 104, 141**)
20 Commercial Blvd.
Novato, CA 94947-6191
Tel: 800-422-7249; Fax: 415-883-3720

American Guidance Service, Inc.
Publishers' Building (**pp. 103, 147, 157, 194–196, 241, 242**)
Circle Pines, MN 55014
Tel: 800-328-2560; Fax: 612-786-9077

The American Occupational Therapy Association, Inc. (**pp. 12, 36**)
4720 Montgomery Lane
PO Box 31220
Bethesda, MD 20824-1220
Tel: 301-652-2682; Fax: 301-652-7711

Cambridge University Press (**pp. 136, 137**)
40 W. 20th Street
New York, NY 10011
Tel: 800-872-7423

Canadian Association of Occupational Therapists (**p. 6**)
110 Eglinton Avenue West, 3rd Floor,
Toronto, Ontario M4R 1A3 Canada

Center for Neurodevelopmental Studies (**p. 38**)
5430 West Glenn Drive
Glendale, AZ 85301

Communication Skill Builders, a division of Psychological Corporation (see below)

Consulting Psychologists Press, Inc. (**pp. 79, 253, 255, 256**)
3803 E. Bayshore Road
PO Box 10096
Palo Alto, CA 94303
Tel: 800-624-1765; Fax: 415-969-8608

Denver Developmental Materials, Inc. (**pp. 122, 123**)
PO Box 6919
Denver, CO 80206

Elbern Publishing (**p. 54**)
PO Box 09497
Columbus, OH 43209
Tel: 614-235-2643; Fax: 614-237-2637

Geri-Rehab, Inc. (**p. 28**)
15 Hibbler Road
Lebanon, NJ 08833

Harcourt, Brace, Jovanovich, Inc. (**p. 187**)
Psychological Corporation
555 Academic Court
San Antonio, TX 78204-2498

Health Sciences Center for Educational Resources (**p. 35**)
University of Washington
T-281 Health Sciences Building
Box 357161
Seattle, WA 98195-7161

Lafayette Instrument Co. (**pp. 153, 160, 161**)
3700 Sagamore Parkway North
P.O. Box 5729
Lafayette, IN 47903
Tel: 800-428-7545; Fax: 317-423-4111

Life Sciences Associates (**p. 26**)
One Fenimore Road
Bayport, NY 11795-2115

Lippincott (**p. 69**)

Mac Keith Press, London.
Obtain from U.S. distributor: Cambridge University Press (see above)

Maddak, Inc. (**pp. 173, 174, 190, 191**)
6 Industrial Road
Pequannock, NJ 07440
Tel: 800-443-4926; Fax: 201-305-0841

McCarron-Dial Systems (**pp. 52, 53, 239, 240**)
PO Box 45628
Dallas, TX 75245
Tel: 214-247-5945

Mind Garden, Inc. (**p. 257**)
P.O. Box 60669
Palo Alto, CA 94306
Tel: 415-424-8493; Fax: 415-424-0475

Model of Human Occupation Clearinghouse (**pp. 13, 14, 63, 64, 78, 220, 221, 226**)

University of Illinois at Chicago

Department of Occupational Therapy (M/C 811)

College of Associated Health Professions

1919 West Taylor Street

Chicago, IL 60612-7250

Tel: 312-996-6901; Fax: 312-413-0256

Modern Curriculum Press (**p. 99**)

13900 Prospect Road

Cleveland, OH 44136

Tel: 216-238-2222

Mosby (**pp. 70, 71**)

National Rehabilitation Services (**pp. 95, 96, 171, 172, 183, 184, 192, 197–200, 202, 204**)

117 North Elm Street

PO Box 1247

Gaylord, MI 49735

Tel: 517-732-3866; Fax: 517-732-6164

NCAST Publications (**pp. 134, 135**)

University of Washington

CDMRC, WJ-10, Seattle, WA 98195

Nelson Canada (sister company NFER-NELSON) (**p. 105**)

1120 Birchmount Road

Scarborough, Ontario

M1K 5G4

Canada

Tel: 800-268-2222; Fax: 416-752-9646

NFER-NELSON Publishing Company Ltd. (**pp. 8, 42, 43, 106, 107**)

Darville House

2 Oxford Road East

Windsor

Berkshire SL4 1DF England

Tel: (0753) 858961; Fax: (0753) 856830

Nottingham Rehab Limited, Nottingham, England (**pp. 97, 98**)

Distributed in the U.S. by: North Coast Medical

187 Stauffer Blvd.

San Jose, CA 95125-1042

Tel: 800-821-9319; Fax: 408-283-1950

Paul H. Brookes (**pp. 73, 74**)

PDP Products (**pp. 90, 162**)

12015 N. July Avenue

Hugo, MN 55038

Tel: 612-439-8865

Pro-Ed (**pp. 62, 100, 163, 164, 231, 232**)

8700 Shoal Creek Boulevard

Austin, TX 78757-6897

Tel: 512-451-3246; Fax: 800-FXPROED

The Psychological Corporation (**pp. 23, 24, 41, 86, 115–117, 121, 125–128, 131, 133, 148, 167, 168, 178, 179, 181, 182, 205, 206**)

555 Academic Court

San Antonio, TX 78204-2498

Tel: 800-228-0752; Fax: 800-232-1223; TDD: 800-723-1318

Psychological and Educational Publications, Inc. (**pp. 108, 109**)

1477 Rollins Road

Burlingame, CA 94010

Tel: 800-523-5775; Fax: 800-447-0907

Raven (**p. 87**)

The Riverside Publishing Co. (**pp. 159, 237, 238**)

8420 Bryn Mawr Avenue

Chicago, IL 60631-9979

Tel: 800-767-8378 or 800-323-9540

Sammons Preston Inc. (**pp. 154, 155**)

PO Box 5071

Bolingbrook, IL 60440-5071

Tel: 800-323-5547; Fax: 800-547-4333

Scholastic Testing Service, Inc. (**pp. 233–235**)
  480 Meyer Road
  Bensenville, IL 60106-1617
  Tel: 800-642-6787; Fax: 708-766-8054

SLACK Incorporated (**pp. 7, 10, 37**)
  6900 Grove Road
  Thorofare, NJ 08086
  Tel: 800-257-8290; Fax: 800-853-5991

Slosson Educational Publications, Inc. (**pp. 142, 143**)
  PO Box 280
  East Aurora, NY 14052
  Tel: 800-828-4800; Tel: Fax: 800-655-3840

S&S Worldwide (**pp. 169, 170**)
  PO Box 513
  Colchester, CT 06415-0513
  Tel: 800-243-9232; Fax: 800-566-6678

Stoelting Co. (**pp. 118, 119, 188, 189**)
  620 Wheat Lane
  Wood Dale, IL 60191
  Tel: 800-860-9775; Fax: 708-860-9775

Thames Valley Test Company, Suffolk, England
  Some tests are distributed in North America by
  National Rehabilitation Services (see above)

Therapy Skill Builders, a division of Psychological
  Corporation (see above)

University of Michigan Press (**p. 124**)
  389 Greene Street
  Ann Arbor, MI 48106-1104
  Tel: 313-764-4392; Fax: 313-936-0456

Western Psychological Services (**pp. 50, 58, 59, 85, 88, 89,
  91, 101, 213, 218, 219**)
  12031 Wilshire Boulevard
  Los Angeles, CA 90025-1251
  Tel: 800-648-8857; Fax: 310-478-7838

Valpar Corporation (**pp. 55, 56**)
  3801 East 34th Street, Suite 105
  Tucson, AZ 85713
  Tel: 800-528-7070; Fax: 520-292-9755

Vocational Research Institute (**pp. 48, 49, 57, 60, 61**)
  1528 Walnut Street
  Suite 1502
  Philadelphia, PA 19102
  Tel: 800-VRI-JEVS

VORT Corporation (**pp. 129, 130**)
  PO Box 60880
  Palo Alto, CA 94306

Index of Assessment Tool Authors

❒ Index of Assessment Tool Authors

Index of Assessment Tool Titles

❏ Index of Assessment Tool Titles

❐ You Can Help

I am interested in hearing about other instruments that are in common use and should be considered for future inclusion in a publication like this. If you are using an evaluation tool that is standardized or uses standard procedures, please let me know. Tear out this sheet and send it to me with any pertinent information about the test, including sample pages or brochures if available. Since occupational therapy practice varies regionally, and this publication is distributed nationally, your contribution can help to improve standards of practice across the country. Thank you for your interest!

TITLE OF EVALUATION:

AUTHOR(S):

SOURCE OR PUBLISHER:

DATE OF PUBLICATION:

COST (estimated; give dollar amount if known):

Tear out this page and send to: Ina Elfant Asher, MS, OTR/L
Thomas Jefferson University
Department of Occupational Therapy
130 S. 9th Street, Suite 820
Philadelphia, PA 19107

[   ]   Please check here if your are interested in information on the Assessments Library at Thomas Jefferson University (beginning Fall 1996).